"Grounded in a modern yet timeless, feminine wisdom-centric, psychospiritual approach. Essential reading for lovers of yoga who are looking for practical yet intuitive methods for integrating Ayurveda into their yoga practice and their lives."

—*Felicia Tomasko, RN, E-RYT, Ayurvedic practitioner, faculty member at Loyola Marymount University and Editor in Chief of* LA YOGA *magazine*

"Dr Siva has written an intelligent, personal and highly practical book for creating a workable Ayurvedic lifestyle. She seamlessly makes this ancient and often esoteric approach to healthcare completely accessible to the modern practitioner—and in the process, allows us to move towards one of the single most important issues facing humans today—healthcare revolution.

Beautifully researched and expressed by Siva's own personal healer's journey, this is a book I will recommend to all of the students who work in my online Ayurveda certification programs. I highly recommend *Ayurveda for Yoga Teachers and Students*—not least for the insights Siva offers on what it means to practice the ancient art of Ayurveda with the type of deep authenticity that true wellness requires."

—*Katie Silcox, New York Times bestselling author of* Healthy, Happy, Sexy – Ayurveda Wisdom for Modern Women

"Start by reading Siva Mohan's introduction to Ayurveda and begin your journey of healing the natural way."

—*Jeffrey Armstrong | Kavindra Rishi, Founder of VASA – Vedic Academy of Sciences & Arts*

"Dr Siva Mohan provides a gift for all readers: a clear, succinct guide to Ayurveda. She demystifies this healing modality without simplifying its insight. Ayurveda provides a pathway to self-awareness and total wellness. Step by step, Dr Mohan explains theory and application in a manner that is universally accessible. Her approach requires no special medicines or herbs, just a willingness to be honest and watchful! Bravo!"

—*Christopher Key Chapple,* Doshi *Professor of Indic and Comparative Theology, Director of Master of Arts in Yoga Studies, Loyola Marymount University, author of* Yoga and the Luminous: Patanjali's Spiritual Path to Freedom

"Siva delivers a focused introduction to Ayurveda lifestyle, guiding readers to be aware of the energetics of their lives, bodies, and emotions. *Ayurveda for Yoga Teachers and Students* is easy to read, well organized, practical, and genuinely helpful."

—*Yogi Cameron Alborzian, bestselling author of* The Yogi Code, The One Plan, *and* The Guru in You

AYURVEDA
for Yoga Teachers and Students

of related interest

Ocean of Yoga
Meditations on Yoga and Ayurveda for Balance, Awareness, and Well-Being
Julie Dunlop
Foreword by Vasant Lad, B.A.M. & S., M.A.Sc.
ISBN 978 1 84819 360 4
eISBN 978 0 85701 318 7

Marma Therapy
The Healing Power of Ayurvedic Vital Point Massage
Dr. Ernst Schrott, Dr. J. Ramanuja Raju and Stefan Schrott
ISBN 978 1 84819 296 6
eISBN 978 0 85701 246 3

Yoga Teaching Handbook
A Practical Guide for Yoga Teachers and Trainees
Edited by Sian O'Neill
ISBN 978 1 84819 355 0
eISBN 978 0 85701 313 2

Ayurvedic Medicine
The Principles of Traditional Practice
Sebastian Pole
ISBN 978 1 84819 113 6
eISBN 978 0 85701 091 9

Ayurvedic Healing
Contemporary Maharishi Ayurveda Medicine and Science, Second Edition
Hari Sharma, MD and Christopher Clark, MD
ISBN 978 1 84819 069 6
eISBN 978 0 85701 063 6

AYURVEDA
FOR
YOGA TEACHERS
AND STUDENTS

BRINGING AYURVEDA INTO
YOUR LIFE AND PRACTICE

SIVA RAAKHI MOHAN, MD, MPH

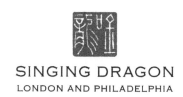

SINGING DRAGON
LONDON AND PHILADELPHIA

First published in 2019
by Singing Dragon
an imprint of Jessica Kingsley Publishers
73 Collier Street
London N1 9BE, UK
and
400 Market Street, Suite 400
Philadelphia, PA 19106, USA

www.singingdragon.com

Library of Congress Cataloging in Publication Data
A CIP catalog record for this book is available from the Library of Congress

British Library Cataloguing in Publication Data
A CIP catalogue record for this book is available from the British Library

ISBN 978 1 84819 393 2
eISBN 978 0 85701 349 1

Printed and bound by CPI Group (UK) Ltd, Croydon, CR0 4YY

Dedication

I dedicate this work to modern yogis looking to feel better, or more whole;

To those needing a life approach that's both healing, and accepting of the fact that we're a bit overwhelmed and depleted;

To those learning to support themselves, in so many ways.

I share this because I love it.

I couldn't do what I love, or be on my path, without you. This is dedicated to your interest in Ayurveda, and in feeling good.

One of my gifts is to show you how to fit Ayurveda into the container of your modern urban life.

And then, use it to change the container entirely.

Wellness is a lifestyle choice.

While this book will walk you through the awareness for well choices, and beginning digestive and emotional health approaches, there is so much more.

Check out my platform to support the foundation of our wellness lifestyle—FoodSexSleep. You'll find online learning, articles, videos, and tools to feel good. The worksheets found in the appendices are also available to download here.

Let's do this together, **Siva**

www.Ayurvedabysiva.com

Acknowledgements

Nikki Estrada for first pushing me to create this curriculum.

Yoga Works for supporting me with ample students and trainings to develop my ideas and test them.

Ayesha Ahmed for reading through the drafts and giving me opinionated, passionate, and spot-on editorial feedback.

Claire Wilson for finding me, and believing in my work enough to advocate for this book.

Lana Shlafer for encouraging me to make this art from the heart.

My mom for feeding me throughout.

My kids for reminding me this doesn't really matter.

Amma for the blessing and mantra that kept my energetics in the right place as I wrote.

My grandma for introducing me to Ayurveda.

The many teachers and authors who have helped to weave the tapestry of Ayurveda and healing and yoga within my body, mind, and spirit.

Contents

Chapter 1

WHY AYURVEDA?

Learning objectives

- Understand the ways in which Ayurveda has been misinterpreted or marketed.

- Get a sense of the different versions of Ayurveda today.

- Glimpse how Ayurveda can interface with yoga.

When I first came to yoga, I felt like it *saved me*. I had blown knees from years of running, terrible posture, was generally self centered and somewhat explosive. It continues to save me from pain in my body, asymmetries and weaknesses, self-destructive tendencies, and frankly, from my own ignorant myopic view of life. I started paying attention to how I operated in life because I was gaining these self-reflective practices on the mat.

Why Ayurveda for yoga teachers?
Custom lifestyle
As you already know, yoga isn't a form of exercise, it's a way of life. I started trying to apply the principles of yoga to my life: ahimsa with vegetarianism, doing 40 day Laxmi mantras for abundance, kitchardi cleanses, and all that other stuff prevalent in modern yoga culture. Some things were helpful, but I felt like I had to abide by all these rules or I wasn't a "yogini."

Generally, however, I still didn't know how to eat, how to handle my emotions, how to make decisions that served my spiritual growth, or how to have healthy relationships. Sometimes, I still don't, but Ayurveda *did* give me these skills. It's just that I forget to use my tools and my awareness. We all do, especially when we're depleted. Ayurveda taught me this, and about my inherent cyclical nature. Its wisdom is like a grandmother, so accepting of who and where we are, and always willing to offer support and a warm cup of something good. This unconditional approach took root within my mind and heart.

Over time, I realized that Ayurveda was the framework from which I learned how to approach my life like one big yoga practice. It's the awareness that allows us to *customize our choices in life,* the way yoga allows us to customize our practice on the mat. Some days you need a few more child poses. Others, you need more breath of fire. Ayurveda was how I learned to be in touch with what I needed that day. The unexpected result of giving myself what I needed more often was healing in all the parts of me.

I'm sure you've felt that yoga has given you this deeper relationship with yourself. And I know that Ayurveda can take you further along that journey, extending the application of everything that yoga teaches us, and *tailoring it to you.*

My journey

Ayurveda is how I started to communicate with my organs, how I started to be able to hear my heart, how I learned to trust my choices, and how I fell in love with my experience of life. I figured out how to be on my dharmic path, prioritized my internal state of harmony, and took back control of my life experience. I changed my career, learned how to feel supported, cleaned up my relationships, cut out drama, and revolutionized how I show up for myself.

Along the way, I remedied my IBS, Hashimoto's thyroiditis, nodulocystic acne, eczema, and chronic sinusitis. Of course it was all related, and being the science dork obsessed with the mind-body connection that I am, I immersed myself in learning *how.* I have an extensive background in health which reveals how invested I am in healing. What I didn't learn in school, but did with my clients and personal journey, is to hold space for your journey to be sacred, no matter what it looks like.

Ayurveda can be complex. It is. It's also simultaneously basic (non-dualism at its best). My goal is to make it simple and enjoyable, so you're more likely to use it. I've come to accept that life doesn't always feel easy, and that Ayurveda can be really effective in helping us feel good even when practiced *imperfectly*. We're always evolving, and we're never going to solve it all, or get it all done—and that's a beautiful relief.

Ayurveda is my practice of staying present with myself and always in touch with, *"Where am I at? What do I need?"* If I can teach you this… Well, I can't. Only your experience, time, and practice can really teach you this. My goal is to open the door, and show you what Ayurveda could *feel* like, to give you the framework and the starting place to begin this practice, and the inspiration to blossom this practice into a way of life.

A dear friend told me, "If it's not something the world needs to hear—something you are burning to share, don't write it." I never doubted this much. What took me so long to finally write this, was that I doubted *myself*. I wanted to have my life and my health in amazing shape before I spread wisdom on *how to do so*. That was rooted in my own fear of not being good enough, or of being criticized for my revolutionary take on a traditional science. It was Ayurveda, again, that allowed me to see that pattern, and to see the healing benefits of showing up for my vision, my voice, my vulnerability, my global impact, my life experience, and my insecure-chubby-little-nerd inner child. Through the Ayurvedic lens, I could see that writing this book was a powerful tool to shift out of my old pattern of insecurity and fear into one of greater self-acceptance. I'll encounter this pattern of self-doubt again, I'm sure. Being able to *see the patterns*, and *knowing what to do* in that particular situation to reach for a healthier pattern, is the core of this lifestyle.

If it's so amazing, why aren't more yoga teachers using Ayurveda?

Every time I begin an Ayurveda workshop for yoga teachers, I ask about the group's previous experience and exposure. Most yoga teachers have heard of Ayurveda. Many have taken a Constitution survey, or a *"dosha quiz."* A decent number have attended an introductory workshop, or had some basics in their 200-hour yoga teacher training (YTT). A handful have worked with a practitioner or read books on their own.

No one feels like they know to *how to apply* Ayurveda to their everyday lives and decisions.

Why is this? Yoga without Ayurveda is like operating on autopilot. It's missing the ability to adjust, to see what is the best kind of yoga for what your *emotional and physical needs are that day*. Ayurveda helps us understand the big picture of how yoga and all its tools play into our day-to-day needs, from mindful eating to sleep-wake rhythms. In other words, Ayurveda is *relevant* to yoga lifestyle, so that's not the issue.

Ayurveda is all around you, even if you haven't noticed yet. We've had access to Ayurvedic herbs and remedies in the West for decades, so access to Ayurveda is not what's lacking. World renowned doctors such as Deepak Chopra and Vasant Lad have been pioneering Ayurveda in the West for decades, with bestselling books, trainings, and videos reaching millions. The increasingly popular field of Functional Medicine has its roots in Ayurveda. You can't miss Ayurveda in the products and marketing in beauty, spa, and nutrition industries. The number of Ayurvedic training programs and schools have grown exponentially outside of India, driven by the popularity of yoga and natural healing systems. In other words, most of us have access to people, programs, and products to be able to learn Ayurvedic lifestyle.

What I'm hearing is that even with access, education, and experience with Ayurveda, it is not being transmitted in a way that allows us to connect to it well—so little is retained or applied. Ayurveda can easily end up seeming like a bunch of esoteric and unrealistic rules on how to achieve an unattainable version of "balance." If you have felt this way, you're not alone.

After surveying hundreds of yoga teachers, the main reasons why they don't feel able to use Ayurveda are:

- it's too abstract

- there are too many rules

- it's too hard to implement in, or doesn't fit well with, modern life

- it's missing the awareness building, so can't modify or individualize

- it's missing the psychospiritutal component, so can't address tough emotions

- it has limited therapeutic benefit (though, only tried short term).

I'd have to agree, and this is how I felt when I first came across Ayurveda. Of course, therapeutic benefit increases when you add in the awareness and emotional components. My goal in this book is to show you how Ayurveda is none of the above. I want Ayurveda to feel simple, applicable, flexible, and self-loving for you, as it does for me, my students, and my clients.

A leading-edge translation
Ayurveda in the West

Largely this oversimplified, rule-based version of Ayurveda is the result of mass marketing, and how Ayurveda has emerged in the modern world. We all understand how mass marketing tends to simplify and dilute concepts. Modern marketing also leans towards quick fixes for low attention spans, which results in what seems like rules to be healthy: *Take this herb to fix X. Eat this way to fix X. Do this morning routine to feel X.*

In the West, Ayurveda has grown as a byproduct of the increasing popularity of a green lifestyle, Eastern Spirituality, Meditation, and Yoga. So, the spiritual components, nutrition, and herbal remedies have been emphasized in the West. This is a stark contrast to the landscape in Ayurveda's birthplace, India.

Effects of colonization

Ayurveda was mostly an underground practice during India's colonization by the United Kingdom. So what was a science transmitted through years of Gurukula (learning organically by being in the presence of a Guru) went underground for hundreds of years.[1] When it re-emerged in newly independent India, it did so in modern Western Medical institutions.[2]

---

1 Saini (2016)
2 "The profound cultural crisis engendered by western technical and material superiority made medicine, like religion and women's status, an important site of constructing cultural and national identity—an endeavor that had to take into account ideas about science, progress, and modernity. Thus, argument for synthesis between the two systems that would preserve the core of the traditional system triumphed over total rejection of either system, for purists envisaged a complete turning back of the clock by returning to a pure Ayurveda and modernists saw no role for Ayurveda in India's triumphal march toward science, progress, and modernity. Just as the various reform movements—in response to the colonial 'gaze'—adopted and adapted western idioms of rationalism, progress, modernity, privileged textual material over customary practices, and attempted to institutionalize traditions through law and the state, the ayurvedic revival movement laid claim to history and science, privileged Sanskritic textual material in keeping with British Orientalism, and fought for state recognition and support." (Ganesan 2010, p.108)

In India, the medical training to become an Ayurvedic doctor is incredibly rigorous, and includes all of Western medical training. Those with a Bachelor of Ayurvedic Medicine and Surgery (BAMS) Degree learn everything we do in the West to get an MD *plus* all the Ayurvedic sutras, herbology, physiology, and body therapies. The science has been overemphasized, and the psychological and spiritual components have been dehydrated out. This is why when a person goes to see an Ayurvedic doctor in India feels very much like visiting an allopathic—within minutes you've been assessed and prescribed.

Effects of patriarchy

Thus, the Western version of Ayurveda is stronger in its humanization and emotional-spiritual approaches and the Indian version has clinical and physiologic superiority. Neither feel quite complete to me. Most importantly, both versions, and all the iterations in between, have a fundamental flaw: the externalization of healing power. We're encouraged to hand over our power to assess and solve for our own healing. I believe this to be an artifact of post-patriarchal layers to healing approaches globally: *Don't trust yourself. Trust the experts, the research, the non-feeling, un-subjective authority figure.*

Modern science has also encouraged the view of the subjective assessment as inferior, or faulty. The search for physical evidence and repeatable results devalued emotional, qualitative, anecdotal, and other forms of sensing and relating energy. As we lost touch with the feminine qualities in our lifestyles, we began to trust and value only quantitative and analytic approaches to energy. Emotions and spirituality became regarded as inferior, weak, and no longer had a place in science.

At this point, you may be thinking that medical expertise and training is required for healing. Yes, there is that. However, you *can* be an expert in the patterns in *your* body and your mind. I've watched thousands of men and women reclaim their power to witness, and respond to these patterns in ways that allow them to heal and thrive. When you step into being the expert on how you feel, the *curendera*, the village *Vaidya*, the midwife, the physician, the yoga teacher all resume the role of *supporting* your healing.

My version of Ayurveda is a *living awareness*. It's science, both quantitative and qualitative. It's steeped in the divine feminine, in realism, in love and acceptance of the human experience, and served with psychospiritual expansion. No artificial flavors, no preservatives, and no "type-yourself-live-this-way" B.S. So dear Reader, I'm pleased to introduce you to my beloved Ayurveda. Even if you've met, my hope is that the way I introduce her is in a way you've never seen her before.

THE EFFECTS OF SUCKING OUT THE PSYCHOSPIRITUAL FROM AYURVEDA

Patriachy **+** Colonization **+** Western mass marketing

Type-yourself-and-live-this-way
Rules
Ayurveda is a physical science
Ayurveda is a sister science to yoga
Hyper-focus on herbs and diet
Allopathicized Ayurveda
Fitting into a Western model

Figure 1.1 *What happened to Ayurveda in the last few centuries*

Summary

- Ayurveda is often misunderstood.

- There is a wide spectrum of how Ayurveda is presented in the West.

- Ayurveda informs Yogic lifestyle.

Chapter 2

WHAT IS AYURVEDA?

Learning objectives

- Be able to define Ayurveda as though you were speaking to a friend.

- Understand how Ayurveda is distinct from modern medicine.

- Understand how Ayurveda is distinct from other natural healing systems.

"The science of life"

Most introductory materials define Ayurveda as "the 5000-year-old science of life." That's not an incredibly illuminating definition. At least, this definition didn't give me a greater understanding of what Ayurveda is. Years later, I get this definition on a deeper level, and I'll try to break it down for you.

Have you ever noticed how many English definitions there are for any Sanskrit word? That's because Sanskrit is a vibrational language. The syllables are chosen to represent energetic states—and there are many ways to describe an energetic state.

Veda means science, and *ayus* means life, or living substance. So we can see where the "science of life" translation comes from. I like to think of it as more the *science of living*; a *lifestyle* that's about optimizing *how good you feel about living*. It's a way to modulate *how good you feel about your experience of life*. It's about *optimizing the living substance* inside of you. These are all various ways to describe a certain approach to feeling damn good in your body, mind, spirit, and life.

Coming from a Western medical perspective, I thought healing systems reveal how to heal, not how to live a great life. With Ayurveda, I realized they are one and the same. I cannot be healthy unless I feel free of internal conflict and stress, in harmony with my inner wisdom and emotions, and with vibrant connection to loved ones and nature. It's all the same journey toward wellbeing.

We cannot separate out the parts of us that are beyond the physical from our physical parts. Because the non-physical parts of us are in deep intimate relationship with our physical body, there is no way to achieve physical health without addressing all of ourselves. All has to feel good: living tissues to life experience to lifestyle.

The "science of life" is such a broad definition. It took me some time to really grasp that Ayurveda *is* so broad—it's a big-picture, healthy lifestyle. It's a system that emphasizes being in tune with yourself so that you are always shifting towards what feels good, in your body and the rest of you.

You can apply this awareness, or approach to anything—so the application *is* broad. Ayurveda uses the same approach to alleviate internal conflict in the emotional body as it does to alleviate digestive symptoms in the physical body.

Ayurveda has become the framework for healing my body, my emotional wellness, and spiritual growth. It's become the way I receive and respond to my life experience, and *now* I can understand why it bears the name "science of life." However, I've found many other ways to define and understand Ayurveda, which may also help you. Since our current context is modern medicine, and we're all likely purveyors of some form of natural healing, I'll reconcile Ayurveda with these approaches as well. Let's take a moment to pronounce it together: ah-yur-vay-dha. (Not ar-yoo-vay-da!)

Holistic healing system

Perhaps foremost, I would define Ayurveda as a holistic approach to healing. I'll define a "holistic healing" system as one that attends to the body, the mind/emotions, and spirit. Holistic healing systems include spiritual growth. The Vedas define spiritual growth as applied awareness. In other words, you grow your self-awareness, and what you need to feel best, and then make decisions accordingly. This inherently grows your consciousness and changes your experience of life.

There are few truly holistic systems. Acupuncture and Chinese herbs would not be a holistic approach without the spiritual process. When practiced with a tie-in to increasing awareness and life choices, acupuncture would be holistic. So, an MD that sells supplements, or a wellness center with a chiropractor, nutritionist, and homeopath would *not* be examples of holistic health approaches.

As you can imagine, having *one* system to be able to address your body, your emotions, your awareness, and your spiritual growth makes things simpler. You have a common platform from which you can view your food, childhood patterns, relationships, or any aspect of your life experience.

With all the studies on stress and psychosomatics in modern medicine, we've proven that emotional states are tied clearly to physical distress. Ayurveda, and all ancient systems, acknowledge that we are more than just our cellular structure, and that to be truly in balance, we must address all of ourselves. While our scientific findings echo this truth, our understanding in the West of how the physical and non-physical parts of us interface is infantile compared to Ayurveda.

Ayurveda and modern medicine

That's a nice segway into a quick comparison of Ayurveda with modern medicine. Modern medicine is our current context of approaching health, and most of us, including myself, use *some* form of it.

Ayurveda views each person as a unique being. We see the variations in the perspectives, the predominant emotional patterns, the digestive patterns, the talents and vulnerabilities, etc. in each of us. We honor that each person's path to disease or symptom and thus their path back to health is also unique. Here, healing is a customized, or individualized, process.

Modern medicine is based on the theory that as we all are the same species, our physiologic workings are the same. Thus each disease has a standardized approach based on the current model of how the disease progresses. With modern medicine, if you come in with a symptom, we have to offer you the same diagnostic tools and treatment options because otherwise we may be faulted (and sued) for not providing equal care to all.

Imagine one person with three weeks of a productive phlegmy cough, which is worse in the morning, and associated with low appetite, increased sleep, and melancholy. Another person presents with a dry hacking cough, which is worse in the evening, and associated with insomnia and anxiety. If they both come in with a chief complaint of "cough," they go through the same standardized medical decision making process, and are likely to receive a similar treatment: a cough suppressant.

Maybe the first case will also get a decongestant and antidepressant, while the second may additionally be offered a sleeping pill or anxiolytic medication. That would only happen if the doctor had enough time to inquire after the person's patterns and associations, emotional states, sleep habits, etc. With the current model of health care, that is, unfortunately, rare. Furthermore, all of these therapeutic options are aimed at symptom relief.

In Ayurveda, these two cases would be approached quite differently, and healing would be customized. Additionally, we would search for the root cause: Why did this cough arise in the first place? What's the state of the immune system? What's happening in this person's life? And then we'd offer some tools for symptom relief, and address the root cause concurrently with symptom alleviation.

As modern medical doctors, we are only trained to offer things that make money—drugs and diagnostic tests. This is the result of the Medical Industrial Complex, and the core reason why many feel unheard and unsatisfied with their modern medical experience. Ayurveda is an off-the-grid sort of system. All of its tools, and even how they are prepared and administered, are based solely on natural elements: herbal preparations, food medicine, routine, decision making shifts, yoga, meditation, and breathwork for example.

As we discussed, Ayurveda is going to involve *everything* in a person's experience. By stark contrast, in modern medicine we have niche specialists and fragmentation. My podiatrist, for example, may never speak with my cardiologist, or endocrinologist, or psychotherapist. Even if they did commune over my overall health, there does not exist in modern medicine a science that details *how* to integrate the knowledge and findings from these various specialists. We are missing the common platform we have in Ayurveda. This fragmentation is a big part of why medical error is the third leading cause of death in the U.S. Death from pharmaceutical and medical interventions is also on the rise.[1]

---

1   Makary and Daniel (2016)

Modern medicine is fantastic for its speed in symptom recovery and handling acute ailments. The trade-off is that many of our tools have side effects. Ayurveda is stronger in tailoring prevention and reversing chronic ailments, but much slower and without side effects. Well, there are some healing "side effects" my clients will note, ranging from "my toenail fungus finally went away," to "I'm yelling at the kids less."

Ayurveda is more work on your part. You sense imbalance; you apply tools. Ayurveda requires a change in your habits. Change requires work. Modern medicine can also suggest changes, but oftentimes we just take a pill or have a procedure. This is an artifact of our modern fast and convenient and "done for you" culture.

Most of us require an Ayurvedic practitioner to help groom our sensing, our choosing of tools, and to teach us the art of tailoring tools. That's true of any new science or lifestyle. Again, it's not in our modern culture to invest in ourselves, and to prioritize how well we feel. Having a doctor take responsibility for care of the ailment, and the insurance take responsibility for payment, fits our modern expectations and health accountability. We can see what results this is producing in our collective modern health experience: increases in mental health ailments, in chronic and degenerative diseases, in cancer, and more people on medication.

I know it may seem like I'm pitching an anti-modern medicine view here. I'm not. I have deep respect for doctors that operate in such a limited and challenging infrastructure. Really, the problems with modern medicine stem mostly from the Medical Industrial Complex, at a level beyond the control of doctors. With my clients, I've seen incredible results for those working simultaneously with both Ayurveda and Western medicine.

Modern medicine is great for treating disease. Ayurveda is for finding health. This subtle, yet important distinction is the reason why the two systems work so well together. Time and time again, we see Ayurveda help decrease recovery time, drug doses, and side effects. The Ayurvedic approach of addressing the root cause supports the healing of chronic ailments in a powerful way, while modern medicine gives us diagnostic tools to monitor healing parameters. One of the great benefits of living in the modern age is our access to so many approaches to healing. Why wouldn't we use all the tools available to us? Ayurveda helps us, eventually, develop an awareness, or intuition on *which tools to use when. And let's not forget that Ayurveda is more than a complement to Western treatment.*

Sadly, the bane of reductionism is so pervasive that is has also quietly crept into the domains of spiritualized systems like Ayurveda. Instead of being seen as a health-promoting system, more and more, Ayurveda is taught, practiced, and promoted worldwide as a complementary system of disease management.[2]

"Mother healing system"

Anthropologically speaking, Ayurveda is considered the oldest healing system known to mankind, and is often referred to as a "mother" of healing systems. In other words, most healing systems can trace their origin and lineage back to Ayurveda. The branches of the multifarious aspects of Ayurveda have developed over time into other healing systems, from Traditional Chinese Medicine to Greek Hippocratic Medicine (which modern Western medicine is derived from).

While Ayurveda is the greater knowledge of what shifts are needed, there are multifarious ways we can accomplish those shifts. Whether we shift energy through Reiki or surgery, Ayurveda understands *what* shifts these different approaches are making, and *why*.

So we are all awed, but why else do we care about this? Well, because this means that we can easily understand other healing approaches from the Ayurvedic perspective. From the Ayurvedic lens, I can understand why my psychotherapist's approaches are good for me at this time, same with my personal trainer; with my chiropractor, etc. I have that *common platform* helping me out once again.

Ayurveda's age also means that Ayurvedic theory and healing approaches have *thousands of years* of observational study to back them up.

What has been happening for a long time, will likely continue.

In modern medicine, we use randomized control trials (RCTs) as our way to study how effective any therapy is, whether that's meditation or a new cancer drug. It's common to find conflicting results on any topic. RCTs are designed based on a premise that all humans are the same, and this is the opposite of the perspective of all the Eastern healing sciences. From Ayurveda's perspective, this is a flawed study design.

---

2   Shunya (2017, p.xiv)

Furthermore, when we do have consistent findings, they leave us with associations more often than producing causal pathways. For example, a study may show that anxiety and IBS are related, but can't elucidate exactly how.

Often what we thought was helpful, on a micro level, is harmful in the big picture. Sunscreen is a good example of this. Once we proved that UV exposure causes skin cancer, we set out to block it. However, the toxicity of the chemicals in sunscreen was completely missed. Epidemiologically, we don't know if the increase in skin cancer rates following the widespread use of commercial sunscreen is due to better screening for skin cancer, or the carcinogens being slathered on in the sunscreen products. We see this with FDA approved food, and beauty products, as well as widely used pharmaceutical drugs, which all had studies prove their effectiveness and safety.

For all these reasons, my opinion is that research is not always trustworthy, and unfortunately, the ways medical studies are financed and statistics are generated play a role in study findings. Personally, I put more faith in an approach supported by thousands of years of observational study, which offers more consistency. Turmeric is anti-inflammatory *every* time. *Pranayama*, or breathwork, has the same physiologic effects across the globe. Yoga benefits *everyone*. Of course, even these tools must be used properly. When tools are meant to be user-customized, instead of standardized, it sometimes makes them safer.

I'm not saying that Ayurveda has the same *results* with all people applying its wisdom. Your results with Ayurveda depend on you and your specifics. What I am saying is that the benefits and approaches of Ayurveda are based on phenomena that have been consistently observed for a long time, and will likely continue.

Now that we've deconstructed the traditional definition, understood it as a holistic healing system, and compared it to other healing approaches, let's get a feel for Ayurveda in our lives.

Pattern mapping system

Ayurveda is a practice of feeling the patterns in our bodies and minds and lives. I often define Ayurveda as a pattern mapping system. Patterns of what? Patterns in eating, patterns in relationships, patterns in poop, patterns in financial stability, patterns in lab results, patterns in back pain—patterns in everything!

Ayurveda provides a language and framework to view the patterns. Once we know the patterns, we can adjust them to have a more balanced, or healthy, experience in life. There are some patterns we want to cultivate for our whole lives; there are others we will naturally battle against our whole lives. We are each unique in the assortment of patterns we are looking to release, or cultivate, in our lives.

From the Ayurvedic perspective, our experiences in life are cyclical, so most of our patterns are recurring. We can even see recurring patterns across generations. We all have patterns. The goal is not to become free of patterns, or symptoms for that matter. That's not the human experience. The patterns are not good or bad. The question we ask when we identify patterns is, "Is this serving my wellbeing at this time?"

Ultimately, all patterns are patterns of energy. How are we going to witness these patterns, and discuss them? We'll discuss this in the next chapter. For now, just understand that the patterns of the major facets of your life determine the patterns in your mind and body. Ayurveda is going to have you look at all those patterns, and make choices based on patterns that feel best, or are balancing.

I'd like to emphasize that conceptually understanding patterns and using the mind to analyze them is just as important as honoring *how we feel* within the various patterns—and this may be a new concept to those that have experienced Ayurveda as a system of rules.

In modern life, we often don't talk about the important things, our deeper patterns, or *how they feel* to us. Imagine two women chatting about a guy who's a romantic prospect. They'll talk about his attributes and what he says or does. It's unlikely that they'll talk about the deeper pattern of what the girl has experienced in love, and whether this experience matches her old pattern or the one she is looking to cultivate. Wouldn't it be cool if they talked about the patterns in how she shows up and responds to relationship dynamics and whether those have served her, or not? About how her patterns reflect those of her parents' relationship, and what patterns she wants to feel?

The same is true for businessmen discussing a deal, parents choosing classes for kids, or deciding what to order for lunch. We look more at surface details of the thing or situation than we do the underlying patterns of *our experience* within situations. Ayurveda has us look at these patterns. It's like you just put on x-ray goggles and see the core patterns in everything in your life. Being able to see your patterns is a part of self realization. At the very least, it helps us to understand why it is we do the things we do.

Awareness

If you have the ability to conceptualize how the various patterns of your life experience are affecting patterns in your body and mind, then you have built a new awareness. I could define Ayurveda as this awareness.

With this awareness, we can make choices to shift patterns. Not only can you use this system to choose diet, routine, activity that is most balancing for your physical body at any given moment; but also to make choices that are most balancing for your emotional state of being.

What this could look like is waking up in the morning, and feeling the patterns in your digestive system—the taste in your mouth, your morning bowel movement, your appetite. Maybe you also feel the patterns in your emotions, in your sleep and level of alertness, in your skin, in your joints. From here, you can choose which foods, activities, herbs, essential oils, people, routine, etc. would be best suited to attend to your patterns and shift them in the direction you'd like to.

It's not about eating Indian food.

Ayurveda offers many tools to shift patterns in the body and mind, but Ayurveda is not the tools themselves. It's the *awareness* of which tools to use and when. A common misperception is that practicing Ayurveda means you have to eat Indian food, take esoteric herbs, or use Sanskrit chants. While Ayurveda was born in India, and so many of its tools are also of Indian origin, the tools to shift patterns are infinite.

Every thing in the natural universe has some healing property in some situation. For example, beer is considered medicinal in the treatment of acute bladder stones because it dilates the ureter, numbs pain, and diureses to flush out the stones. Here, the use of beer is Ayurvedic. The use of an ice pack, a warm salt bath, making love, an essential oil, the color purple, expressing something long withheld, are all Ayurvedic *if they are being chosen with the awareness* of how they will shift a pattern in the direction we want to head.

Empowerment process

There is no cookie-cutter approach to healing. There is no diet or herbal supplement that will be balancing to all of us, all of the time. Further, we're going to need a multifaceted approach to attend to the many aspects of each one of us.

With this avalanche of alternative health options, we can find someone that benefited, and research to either support, or negate, the benefit of *any* supplement or health approach. Great, so how do you choose which is best for you and how do you evaluate if it continues to be good for you as you change? Well, once you develop the awareness of what patterns are present in your life, and how they affect you and your health, you'll have a system to choose by.

In other words, I could also define Ayurveda as the application of this awareness, or the practice of *choosing what is best for you* in any given moment. Knowing how to choose what is best for you is empowerment, and so I can also view Ayurveda as an empowerment process. It's a lifestyle in which you consciously choose the energetics of your life.

Once you learn to plug into the energetics of your choices, decision making feels more clear and easy. Only you are in the experience of your body, your feelings, and your life. So really, only you are in the position to really choose what feels best for you.

I love acupuncture. I love chiropractic, homeopathy, Reiki, etc. Every healing modality offers great value. However, I have to keep going to the acupuncturist, or practitioner, to use the tools they have. With Ayurveda, I learn how to use tools for myself. Even the tools I use, and how I use them at various times, are tailored to me.

As humans going through this life thing together, we need each other. We need support and insight from people. That used to be elders and healers, and now it's therapists and life coaches. In modern life, we subscribe to a lot of fear-based approaches, and obviously our wellbeing can generate a lot of fear. So we reach for doctors, or practitioners, or experts and research. And in the process, we disconnect from our own wisdom and intuition about what is happening with us.

The moment I go to a practitioner, I hand over my power to heal myself, and say, "Please, practitioner, figure out what's going on with me, and solve it." No matter how sophisticated the practitioner or doctor, their assessment cannot beat the first-hand expression of my body and my emotions that I feel. The problem is that we've turned off dialogue with our bodies, and deep feeling. That's okay. Working with healers is great, and often necessary. But, *our insight* has to be a key part of the diagnostic and remedial process for it to be accurate and truly healing.

Imagine that practitioner was sharing their insight and listening to you and collaborating with you to elucidate the patterns, and then holding your hand through implementing healing approaches, educating you and empowering you all the while.

With the education and support, you learn how to see and address your unhealthy patterns, and at some point you don't really need the practitioner on a regular basis anymore. You've got the awareness. You know what's going on and why. You've got some tools to use when you do the things you do that lead you to feel the way you feel.

This is an empowerment based model of healing, and I'm pioneering this model of Ayurveda. What you feel and think about your health matters, and only you can make the changes in your life to make the shifts that are needed for health.

The hardest part of Ayurveda is trusting yourself.

We're not accustomed to feeling. We're not taught to trust our own assessment. Yet over and over again, people are feeling that something is off that the doctors can't explain. Others are experiencing wellness despite what the doctors say is possible. In this empowered model of Ayurveda, we don't lose sight of how you feel, and building your awareness of the factors that affect how you feel is the most important goal of the journey. As I walk clients through this process, their greatest challenge, and mine in my own healing journey, is trusting ourselves.

It just takes time to get more connected with our inner guidance system. In the beginning my clients will come in and ask me what I think, and depend more on my suggestion. Within a few months of validating them, they come into greater assurance of their own wisdom. It starts out as "I don't know. What do you think Dr. Mohan?" and then shifts to "Well, I was feeling and thinking this, and what do you think Dr. Mohan?" and then to "I felt this, so I chose this and and I thought of you as I made those shifts." It's so exciting to see client after client connect to their inner "GPS." Ayurveda can be a way to connect with your inner guidance system, a way to learn to listen to yourself. All we need is time, support, and consistent practice.

Summary

You can now define Ayurveda! Ayurveda can be viewed as:

- a healing approach that includes spiritual growth

- a platform to view the patterns in your body and mind, and how they are related to the patterns in your life

- an awareness of what is best for you at any given moment, based on how it modulates your patterns

- an empowered, conscious lifestyle.

As you can see, there are so many ways to understand Ayurveda. Every experience of Ayurveda is a personal one. At this point, you have a background in the traditional definitions of Ayurveda, as well as a nontraditional insight into what Ayurveda *could* be.

Ultimately, Ayurveda is a system to feel good. I don't mean the kind of superficial "feel good" after some wine, or a momentary "feel good" such as eating a clean, organic, nourishing meal. I mean a deep connected and aware feel good about the energetics of your life. In the next chapter, we'll begin looking at *how* we can start to identify patterns.

Chapter 3

EVERYTHING IS ENERGY

Fundamental Tenets of Ayurveda

Learning objectives

- Be able to conceptualize the *doshas*.

- Begin to tune into qualities of energy.

- Glimpse an energetic perspective of your life.

Our learning objectives in this chapter are threefold. First we want to get you familiar with the primary units of energy categorization—the *doshas*. Next, we want to have you be able to start to feel or sense the qualities around you, and in your life.

Energetic patterns

We've just answered what Ayurveda is, and now we'll expand on one of the fundamental philosophies underlying Ayurveda, and all ancient science: *everything is energy*. Because the world is just one big soup of energy, everything is interconnected. Just as a storm in Asia can affect the weather in California, an energetic shift in your life can affect your mind and your body.

In this chapter, we'll focus on the basics to be able to witness energetic patterns. Eventually, this skill will help you to make choices that are energetically beneficial for your wellbeing. I'll introduce the basic energy categorization system of Ayurveda: the famous five elements and three primary energy types. We'll then touch on how to begin figuring out the energetics of you and various aspects of your life.

Everything in this universe can be reduced to the same thing: energy. You. Me. Food. Climate. Quantum physics, chemistry and biology all are based on this same tenet. Although we're taught that the study of energy is modern science, understanding of the natural universe was actually very sophisticated in ancient cultures around the globe. In the Vedic period in India, for example, they were measuring the speed of light through various substances without labs, or high tech microscopes. Furthermore, ancient cultures expressed energetic patterns in ways people could relate to.

It's quite moving to appreciate that all ancient cultures had energetic awareness as the core of their understanding of the natural universe. Every science and art from every ancient culture was about observing and modifying energetic patterns in nature, and in our lives, bodies, and hearts.

E=mc², and E=love.

Everything that has molecules is energy in modern science, but ancient sciences also studied and honored subtle energetics. Take love for example, it cannot be measured, and neither can attention, or intention. But we can sense all of these. Ayurveda has a vast and sophisticated understanding of subtle energy. That's beyond our scope in this book, but this is my area of interest and I have a lot of articles on my website related to emotions and mindsets. For our purposes here, I want to make the point that feelings, and things you can feel but can't measure, are also energy.

Categorizing energy

As I mentioned earlier, Ayurveda is a game of pattern mapping. Categorizing helps us to understand patterns. Like any broad topic, there are ways to break it down and categorize it. This aids in discussing and understanding the subtleties. We want to be able to categorize energy so we can see patterns, talk about them, be more aware of the energetics of our lives and how they affect us.

Once we get a sense of what kinds of patterns are coming in, and how they are affecting us, we can begin to shift them. In Ayurveda, we find the existing patterns that are not serving us, and cultivate new patterns which are more balancing for us. We'll discuss balancing more in Chapter 6.

Modern science breaks down the broad phenomenon of energy into atoms, as described by the periodic table of elements and via molecular structure. The periodic table of elements is not a very useful categorization system because it is not easy to use or relate to, or accessible to most. I can't *sense* different types of atoms. Even if I send something into a lab to have its atomic composition determined, I have no way of using that information. Furthermore, I cannot determine the energetic breakdown of anything that is not a physical entity: color, emotion, texture, sound, for example.

Thankfully, there are many ways to categorize any phenomenon. Let's take our closets as an example of this. We all have clothing, and everyone's closet is categorized in their own unique way. Some may organize by color. Others by season. Others by garment type. For each of us, the most important thing is that the categorization system we are employing in our own closets makes sense to us. Any categorization system has got to be intuitive for the user in order to be useful. Think of your favorite app—if it's easy to use, you'll use it more. The *doshas* may not start out as a categorization system that feels intuitive, but they can be over time.

I think of getting to know the *doshas* like getting to know friends. There are traits and descriptions and impressions we have when we meet someone. After a year of getting to know them, we have a good feel for them. As you spend more time identifying the *doshas* in yourself and your life, you'll get a better intuitive feel for them. Once you get a feel for categorizing energy, you can't really turn it off. Just like when you get to know someone, even if you spend some time away from them, you still have a feeling of them—you don't just un-get-to-know them.

Color analogy

The way we understand color is a great example for how Ayurveda looks at categorizing energy. There are millions of colors. We organize them first into color families: reds, oranges, yellows, etc. We can further reduce down to the level of the three primary colors: red, yellow, and blue. All colors are a combination of the three primary colors. *Millions* of colors each have their own ratio of the three primary colors.

In Ayurveda, we categorize the entire Universe of energy first into the five elements of nature: earth, water, air, space (aka ether), and fire. The Vedic sages described everything in their lives in the terms of the five elements, from food to personalities.

Just like we get more specific about a color when we know its ratio of red, yellow, blue; we get more specific about energy when we describe the ratio of the three primary energies. These three primary energies are called *doshas*.

Doshas may be the only Sanskrit word I really use in this book, because it's so much simpler than saying "primary energy." I'm going to focus our study at the level of the three primary energies, or *doshas*, because this is our most direct path to applying Ayurveda in our own lives. I want to keep this as simple and effective as possible, so you'll use it.

Color	Energy
Color Family	Five elements
Primary Color (RYB) Ratio	Primary Energy (VPK) Ratio

The 5 elements and 3 *Doshas*

So let's get into categorizing energy Ayurveda style, starting with a brief review of the five elements. The five elements are not literal. For example, the element *water* represents an energy that is fluid, absorbing, nourishing, cooling, flowing, moist. If a relationship is flowing and nurturing, we can say that the energetic exchange between the two people has a good amount of "water energy." We don't mean literally that there is water between them.

If you think about it, all words are representations of energy.

Even though we don't have a robust modern language to describe energy the way all ancient cultures did, our idioms do have some remnants of acknowledging the qualities of the five elements, for example, *cold* shoulder; *fiery* temper; Mother Earth; *air*-head; *dry* conversation; *icy* stare.

Chart 3.1 outlines the qualities of the five elements, as taught in traditional Ayurveda. I *don't* think this is very helpful, as these are not the words with which we describe our lives. In the bottom row, are some of my own adjectives to describe the qualities of the five elements as I feel them. This is just to show you that you can use your own words and still use this categorization system.

Chart 3.1 Qualities of the five elements

Element	Ether	Air	Fire	Water	Earth
Traditional qualities	light soft smooth subtle	cold dry rough mobile	hot sharp oily	heavy oily wet cold	heavy stable hard dense
Additional qualities (adjectives)	ethereal floating ephemeral transparent	animating fresh invigorating enthusiastic	intense illuminating catabolic discerning	fluid absorptive nourishing flowing buffering	fertile sturdy solid protective maternal

Vedic sages used the categorization system of the five elements, because they lived in and had an intimate relationship with nature at that time. This made the five elements an intuitive categorization system *back then*. These days, not many of us have an intimate relationship with the five elements.

We don't live in nature. When I ask people for words to describe the five elements, the descriptions are rather simple, like describing fire as "hot." It's not until you really spend a lot of time getting to know fire that you may describe it as "discerning," or "digestive." It's only after a lot of practice that I can estimate how much of the elements are in a couch, a drink, a Powerpoint presentation, or a person. If the elements are too abstract for you, *don't use them*. They are not necessary to practice Ayurveda. We can just focus on the three primary energy types as the energy categorization system in that case.

The reason Ayurveda typically begins with the five elements is because we then introduce the three *doshas* in the terms of the elements. For example, one of the *doshas* is like fire. Another is like water and earth. Another is like wind, or air and ether combined. This approach is similar to being better able to conceptualize a primary color ratio when you know which color family it's in.

The elements are here to help understand the *doshas*. So, if they serve you, use them. If you easily associate "hot" with fire and that helps you to be able to get to know Pitta energy, great. That's how understanding the elements can help with understanding the *doshas*. If not, set your focus on understanding the three *doshas*, and you'll be fine. Remember, if you cannot relate to the descriptive approach, you're unlikely to use it. I'm going to teach you how to get to know the *doshas* in a more big-picture way as well.

The 3 doshas

Vedic sages noticed that the five elements were often found in combination. With this observation, they were able to simplify the categorization system to three primary energy types.

In Chart 3.2, I've included the traditional description of the qualities of these three primary energies. Once again you can see they are not the words we typically use to describe things. For now, I just want to emphasize how the qualities of the *doshas* are the same as the elements that combine to form them.

Chart 3.2 *Doshas* described by the qualities of their elements

Elements	Ether	Air	Fire		Water	Earth
Dosha	Vata		Pitta		Kapha	
Qualities	dry light cold subtle clear mobile dispersing astringent bitter		hot sharp light oily pungent sour spreading		heavy slow cool oily damp smooth soft static viscous sweet	

Now, I'm going to present the *doshas* in a more big-picture way. Close your eyes for a moment, and just relax your forehead, and take a deep breath. Here is what the three primary energy types *feel* like to me:

- Kapha is a still, stable, growing, attached, protective, grounded, fertile, creating kind of energy. It's the energy of the womb, moist earth, and springtime.

- Pitta is a doing, producing, efficient, cutting to the core, sharp, confident, clear, logical, working kind of energy. As fire digests wood into light and heat, Pitta is an energy that breaks things down, and turns them into what is needed.

- Vata is a moving, changing, cold, dry, reactive, unattached, light kind of energy. Like the wind, ever moving and unpredictable. Like the wind, it's stimulating, but depleting. The wind erodes mountains.

I once had a pandit tell me a joke. He asked me what GOD stood for, and then chuckled and did the Indian head bob as he revealed that GOD was an acronym for Generating, Operating, and Destroying, as these are the three primal forces. I thought to myself, "aha, Kapha, Pitta, and Vata!" I hope that no one is too offended by my pandit acronym, and maybe it will help you remember the essence of Kapha, Pitta, and Vata in a big-picture perspective.

It makes sense. Everything is generated, functions, and then degenerates. We can see how these three types of energy are the basis of all things from planets to cells. Everything in the natural Universe is created, does some function, and then goes away—the cycle of life.

- Kapha is the generating/ creating energy.
- Pitta is the operating/ functioning energy.
- Vata is the degenerating/ entropic energy.

Chart 3.3 *Doshas* and big-picture definition

Element	Ether	Air	Fire	Water	Earth
Dosha	Vata		Pitta	Kapha	
Qualities	*Degenerating*		*Operating*	*Generating*	
	Wear and tear		Does the work	Puts together	
	Erratic		Productive	Maternal	
	Movement		Transformation	Support	

Doshas are inseparable

If we look at your computer or phone as an energetic organism from the Ayurvedic perspective, we could see Vata in the movement of the keypad or your finger on the touchscreen, Pitta in the software code that really accomplishes all the tasks, and Kapha as the infrastructural hardware that provides the stable foundation for all this to occur.

In every human cell, I find Kapha in the protective fatty cell membrane and moist cytoplasm. I find Pitta energy in the enzymes at work and the processes of transcription and translation. Vata energy allows for all the movement within the cell from the unraveling of the DNA, to the movement of vesicles.

Let's play this game with an organ system. In digestion, Kapha energy is in the saliva that coats and moistens the food, and in the protective mucus lining of the stomach and the colon. Pitta energy is in the digestive enzymes, and stomach acid, breaking the food down and transforming it into macronutrients. Vata energy allows us to move the food down the digestive tract, to move nutrients across cells for absorption, and to move undigested matter out.

The *doshas* are in everything. Everything is made up of energy. We sense energy by the qualities we feel. We rarely sense one quality in isolation. In fact, most everything has some combination of qualities, including us. Just as we rarely see pure red, yellow, and blue, we rarely see pure Vata, Pitta, or Kapha. More often we see a blend of colors.

I can eat soup that has many qualities—creamy, spicy, earthy, heavy, and slightly sweet. Even though it may have many qualities, it will have some that are the most predominant in *my experience* of eating it, and those are the *doshas* I'm taking in the most of when I eat the soup. Similarly, our experience of our relationships, our food, our routine, and our work may have mixed qualities. The qualities we feel the most in *our experience* of any facet of our lives will reveal the *dosha*(s) we are taking in through those aspects.

We're going to practice identifying the *doshas* in a moment. For now, I want to re-emphasize how amazing it is to be able to describe everything happening in your life, in your body, and in your emotions with the *same language*; with the same categorization system. This common platform allows us to see how our lives are affecting us.

Sensing energy
Identify doshas by qualities

I can describe anything in terms of these three primary energies, Vata, Pitta, and Kapha (VPK). And so can you! How? Simply by identifying the qualities present in anything. If you are feeling that quality, you are taking in that *dosha*.

If the quality of the dosha *is there, the* dosha *is there.*

Remember, it's going to be some time before you have an intuitive feel for the *doshas*. Your relationship with Vata, Pitta, Kapha will get better and better over time. In the meantime, I created a tool for you to start to identify the *doshas* in your life: *Qualities of VPK Chart*.

In this *Qualities of VPK Chart* (Chart 3.4), I list many qualities of Vata, Pitta, and Kapha. Up top, I have the traditional descriptions of their qualities. Few of us would use these words to describe how our lives feel. So, I've put together a long list of qualities in my own words, that you may be able to better relate to. This is not an all inclusive list of every word to describe VPK—that's impossible. These are qualities of the *doshas*, as I've experienced them. Over time, I'm sure you'll have your own words too.

I tried to include words that describe routines, relations, and food. My hope is that you can feel one of these qualities in whatever you are assessing, and then sense from the chart whether V, P, or K are present. Post a copy somewhere you can see it regularly, like on your phone, your fridge, or the office corkboard. After about two weeks of looking at it occasionally, you'll have a good part of it memorized. Plus, it's a great conversation starter.

Chart 3.4 Qualities of VPK chart

Dosha	Vata	Pitta	Kapha
Traditional qualities	dry light cold subtle clear mobile dispersing astringent bitter	hot sharp light oily pungent sour spreading	heavy slow cool oily damp smooth soft static viscous sweet
Additional adjectives	scattered irregular hard ungrounded effusive flaky restless unsubstantial animating fresh floating invigorating empty ethereal open vast crunchy unpredictable unexpected vibrant depleted crisp enthusiastic ephemeral transparent unstable fast	intense critical discerning pure passionate penetrating transformative processing to-the-point digesting analyzing strategizing working illuminating catabolic fluid flowing bright glowing tart spicy acidic tangy stinging burning producing evaluating	dense regular thick grounded calm unchanging still substantial dull full cluttered unprocessed slimy held absorptive buffering nourishing fertile sturdy solid protective maternal moist foggy clouded unclear nurturing

Remember, the energetic composition (VPK) of anything can be understood by sensing its qualities. So, when you note these qualities in anything, you are sensing the presence of Vata, Pitta, and Kapha.

- Notice there are some words that may seem more "good" or "bad" because we are conditioned to categorize the world this way. For example, depleted may seem like a "bad" aspect of Vata, and sweet may seem like a "good" aspect of Kapha. In reality, the designation is in our minds, and relative to the beholder.

- What may be intense to me, for example, may not seem intense to you. This could be the case if I had a sensitive (more Vata) nature/ Current State, or if you had more accepting (more Kapha) of a nature/Current State.

- That we perceive differently underscores our unique nature, or Constitution. We'll go into this in Chapter 4.

- Each *dosha* has its beneficial qualities, which are augmented *when we are in balance* in that *dosha*. Similarly, each *dosha* has its detrimental qualities, which we see when we have imbalance. We'll explore this concept further in Chapters 5 and 6, while looking at your Current State and defining imbalance.

You are made to sense energy

The adjectives you use in describing any energy input in your life (relationship, job, climate, food) is essentially a list of the qualities of energy you are taking in. By identifying the qualities of energy, we can more easily connect to which *dosha* is present.

We don't need anything to be able to describe how something feels. *We just need to feel.* In modern life, we've turned off a lot of our feeling and sensing skills in favor of our analytical and cognitive abilities. Like anything in the body, if you don't use it, it atrophies. On the bright side, the more we flex our ability *to sense and describe what we are feeling*, the stronger it becomes.

You can do this, and you'll get better at it over time. Here are your three clear steps for starting to see the world through Ayurveda:

1   *Feel* the qualities present.

2   Identify the *dosha* related to that quality, using your chart as a tool at first.

3   Feel the *doshas*. Over time, start to remember which qualities are associated with the *dosha*.

Just like learning anything new, it's analytical and cerebral at first, but can then become intuitive. Remember how awkward and terrifying it was to make a turn across oncoming traffic when first learning to drive? Over time, you don't even think about it—you just do it naturally.

We have many automatic sensory receptors, to feel all kinds of energetic shifts within ourselves. We can all feel more than our five main senses, such as when someone is staring at us from behind. We may not be able to consciously tap into our blood vessels sensing minute variations in blood pressure, but the body senses it and responds without our awareness. Similarly, your body and emotional body are sensing and responding whether you are tapped in or not. Once you do start to become aware of what it's sensing and how it's responding, you can work with your body and mind on the same page.

Let's practice identifying the *doshas* in both tangible things, like food and climate, and some less tangible things, like experiences and interactions. In the chart below, you can see the qualities present in the examples and the *doshas* that are related to those qualities.

Chart 3.5 Examples of identifying qualities and *doshas*

Example	Qualities / Adjectives	Dosha
A sunny day in Southern California	hot, sunny, bright, consistent	P
	dry, desert wind	V
An unhealthy relationship	aggressive, judgement, anger intense (heat)	P
	unstable, extremes (movement), lack of intimate connection (unanchored)	V
Indian restaurant food	spicy-hot, warm	P
	moist, heavy, nourishing	K

Qualities are relative to the observer

What may be spicy hot to me may not be to you. What may feel intense to one person may not to another. When we assess the energetic impact on someone, we have to accept how things feel to *that* person. Ayurveda is *always* from the point of view of the person being assessed. Only you can describe how something feels to you.

At the same time, there are situations in life that bring in a lot of a certain energetic for all of us. For example, aggressive athletic training will increase Pitta for everyone participating, as all the athletes are taking in more Pitta with the training.

Chart 3.6 Different situations with the same qualities can bring in the same *dosha*

Example	Qualities / Adjectives	*Dosha*
Having just lost a job	Undefined ungrounded void (ether) lacking unexpected	V
New mother	Emptying (womb and milk); depleting; erratic sleep	V
Post-menopausal / andropausal stage of life	dry light stiff fragile depleted degenerating letting go transition	V

The energetics of life experiences can be assessed. Getting laid off is a process that involves a great deal of Vata. Even if it ends up being the best thing for you, the experience has the qualities of uncertainty, insecurity, lack of definition, ambiguity, void, and transition. These are all qualities of Vata.

Relationship energetics can be assessed in the same way. A new mother's affect toward her newborn can be overflowing with Kapha energy. For the baby, it's a Kapha input. For the mama, however, all her loving care for baby is a net depletion, or Vata experience. Indeed, even though she may be overjoyed, postpartum women commonly have high Vata symptoms such as anxiety, dryness, constipation, low immunity, hypersensitivity, big emotional swings, and light sleep.

Even experiences such life stages can be assessed. After our fertility ends, we enter a high Vata stage of life. This is why so many elderly go through symptoms of high Vata such as thinning tissues, dryness, constipation, low appetite, fatigue, light sleep, low bone density, and easy overwhelm, to name a few.

These are three very different high Vata energy experiences. *How* we bring in Vata, Pitta, and Kapha will all be unique to our life story.

Fear, insecurity, indecisiveness, fleeting thoughts, anxiety, and inability to concentrate are all evidence of high Vata in the mind and nervous system, and it's no coincidence that these feelings often accompany a high Vata experience. So even though they are very different ways to be bringing in a lot of Vata, all three of these cases in the chart above could be experiencing very similar symptoms.

Summary

- Everything in the universe is energy.

- Categorizing energy helps to understand patterns.

- The three primary energy types are Vata, Pitta, Kapha (VPK).

- The energetic composition (VPK) of anything can be understood by sensing its qualities.

- Energy taken in is relative to what the observer feels.

So, to review, everything in our universe is a form of energy. To better understand ourselves and our experience of being in this universe, we can look at energetic patterns. Categorizing energy allows this deeper discovery into patterns of energy within and around you. In Ayurveda, we categorize all the forms of energy as some combination of three primary energy types, or *doshas*: Vata, Pitta, Kapha. To sense these three primary energies, we simply need to use our senses and observe *the qualities present.*

The reason any of us are drawn to learn about a healing science is so we can apply what we've learned to our own lives. Indeed, this is our homework for this chapter. In the *VPK in my Life Worksheet* (Appendix 1), you are going to identify the *doshas* present in four major aspects of your life: work, routine, a main relationship, and food. The worksheet has detailed directions, but essentially we'll use the adjectives and qualities in our reference chart to complete the worksheet. To summarize your findings:

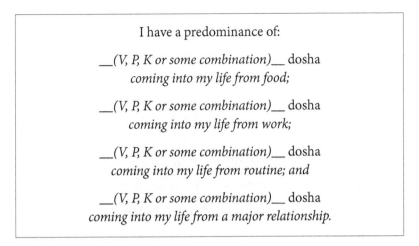

You've made it through the fundamentals of Ayurveda! In the next two chapters, we are going to shift the focus to you. We'll explore VPK in your Constitution and your Current State of health.

Chapter 4

YOUR UNIQUE NATURE

Constitutions, Why They Matter,
How to Use Them

Learning objectives

- Be able to define Constitution.

- Understand what Constitution determines about you.

- Get a sense of your own Constitution.

- Understand the limitations of a Constitution-centered approach.

Now that we are beginning to sense VPK around us, our next step is to look at the VPK *within* ourselves. In this chapter, we'll explore the concept of Constitutions and end with a survey to assess your own Ayurvedic Constitution. So, our learning objectives are to understand Constitution and what it tells you about yourself. Also, I'd like you to get a sense of your own Constitution while keeping in mind the limitations of a Constitution assessment.

In the last chapter, we learned a primary tenet of Ayurveda: everything is energy. A second fundamental tenet is that we are all born with a unique energetic composition, often called a "Constitution." We each have Vata, Pitta, and Kapha; however, the ratio to which we carry and express these energies varies with individuals. Your Constitution describes the primary energetic ratio you were created with. Everything has a Constitution, or VPK ratio. Just like every color has a red:yellow:blue ratio, your Constitution is your personal ratio of VPK.

We aren't created equally; rather, artfully, each with our own hue.

While each being is an individual manifestation of energy, we are still all made of the same stuff. For this reason, it's relatively easy to find patterns and commonalities between people, processes, and environments.

There is no perfect or ideal Constitution, just like there is no perfect color. Every Constitution has its own gifts, and *all* have challenges. So you don't get to look at your Constitution and judge it as good or bad.

Where does my Constitution come from?

So how is our Constitution formed? Well, it comes from our biological parents. Imagine we've got three big barrels, one each for Vata, Pitta, and Kapha. Your mom poured in the levels of VPK she had at that moment of conception, and then dad did the same. The resultant levels are your unique ratio, or Constitution.

The energetics of mom's pregnancy experience also play a role, modulating how the DNA is expressed. For all our modern variations in conception, baby's Constitution is still going to be based on the current energetic state of the egg and sperm donors combining, and still modulated by the woman's energetic experience while carrying the embryo.

Notice I did not say mom and dad simply combine their Constitutional ratios, it's based on their energetic state in that *moment*, or Current State. We'll go into Current State in next chapter. In the meantime, let's simply understand that the differences among biological siblings are due to the difference in where the parents were energetically at the time of conception and mom's pregnancy experience. We share the same DNA with biological siblings, but how that DNA is expressed can be so varied. This is the study of Constitutions, which relates to the modern science of epigenetics.

When I was conceived, my parents were in a high VP state. They were new immigrants, hustling, and with a good deal of transition (V), scarcity (V), hard work (P), and intensity (P). The pictures of them at that time show a thin, fit, stylish couple with intense expressions on their faces. Indeed, I have a lot of VP in my Constitution. Five years later, when my sister was conceived, they were settled—mom was a housewife, dad was in management, they owned a car and a home. In the photographs around this time, they are overweight, laughing, holding each other, and usually surrounded by friends. All of this translates to them having a lot more Kapha qualities in their lives. My sister's Constitution reflects this energetic change in their lives, and she has much more K than I do. When you look at us, you can see I have more VP and less K than she does. This helps to explain why my body and mind express more VP traits and tendencies, while hers expresses more K ones, from the same parental DNA.

What your Constitution reveals

Now that we know how you got your Constitution, let's explore what it tells us about you. There are three main things your Constitution determines about you. The first is your body structure, the second your default emotional patterns, and the third your tendencies towards ailments.

In the physical body, your Constitution will govern things like your size, shape, pigmentation, and physical tendencies (like muscle tone). Of course all of these are changeable *to an extent*. You can greatly shift your muscle tone by working out. However the degree to which your body is likely to be muscularly toned is still governed by your Constitution. I can go to the gym and work twice as hard to see the same muscle tone as a friend who has more Pitta in her Constitution, and thus greater muscle tone in her nature.

No matter how much I exercise, I won't change how tall I am, or how wide my hip bones are. I may change my tan with sun exposure, but without actively tanning, there is a normal level of pigmentation that my body will keep heading toward as a baseline. In other words, your Constitution determines your set point and defines the *default settings* in your body.

Second, your Constitution determines your default emotional patterns. This is similar to the concepts of childhood defense mechanisms or core personality traits in the West. I think of this as how you innately *receive and respond* to life. In general, you would see your Constitution-based personality traits early in life, before too much imbalance has set in. Even in babies, we can see Constitutional tendencies in personality with how they nurse, relate, sleep, and digest.

The third thing a Constitution determines is what kinds of tendencies we have for imbalance. Our Constitution reveals inherited disease tendencies and vulnerable tissues. We all have patterns and tendencies towards disease. With the understanding of our Constitutions, we can better understand which tendencies we have and why.

In general, folks with a lot of:

- V are challenged with Vata ailments; Vata symptoms involve degeneration and irregularity

- P are challenged with Pitta ailments; Pitta symptoms involve heat, infection, and inflammation

- K are challenged with Kapha ailments, like accumulation and stagnation.

There can be combinations too. Someone with a lot of two *doshas* will have a propensity towards imbalance in both of those *doshas*. Someone with roughly similar amounts of VPK has about equal probability of VPK imbalance.

Additionally, there are bodily organs associated with each *dosha*. When we have a lot of a *dosha*, the organs associated with that *dosha* are areas of vulnerability for us. These are areas of the body in which the *dosha* is said to "reside" and build up. For example, the skin is an organ that is associated with Pitta. Someone with a lot of Pitta in their Constitution is more prone to have Pitta symptoms in a Pitta organ, like acne or rash. Another example is the Vata in the pelvic bowl area: those with a great deal of Vata in their Constitution will commonly experience Vata symptoms in the pelvic bowl such as low back pain, gas, bloating, constipation, and menstrual cramps.

So, your Constitution really does affect your experience of health. But it's not set in stone. The Constitution defines your *defaults, vulnerable areas, and tendencies.* To me, Constitutions help me define the *probability* of patterns occurring. Then, I can pre-empt those patterns. By understanding our Constitution patterns, we can tailor a healthy lifestyle of prevention. In fact, the vast majority of Ayurvedic approaches are preventive in nature. Even curative approaches are imbued with preventive measures.

It's really all about understanding who you are, what you are likely to experience, and working to balance those patterns. In order to get you ready to take a look at your Constitution, let's review a few basics and clarify a few common misperceptions.

Doshic predominance

One of the most common responses I hear when I share that I'm in the field of Ayurveda is, "Oh, I think I'm a Vata." No one is a Vata. Or a Pitta for that matter. We are all VPK, in varying ratios.

If you have a significantly greater amount of one *dosha* in your ratio, we say your Constitution is "predominant" in that *dosha*. You will easily see the qualities of this *dosha* in your physical make up and personality. In the charts below, I model three examples of Constitutional ratios.

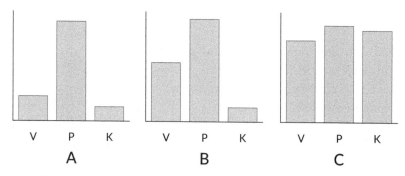

Figure 4.1 *Various forms of doshic predominance; all Pitta predominant*

In our Constitutional energetic ratio, we can have a *dosha* that is predominant. Example A shows a single doshic predominance. You can see that person A has much more Pitta than Vata and Kapha. We would call this "Pitta predominant," and expect to see a lot of Pitta qualities in this person.

The majority of us have two *doshas* in greater ratio to the third, and this is called "dual-doshic predominance" Example B shows a Pitta-Vata predominant Constitution. This means that we will see mostly a combination of these two doshic qualities in person B's body and persona.

There are fewer of us that have the three *doshas* in approximately equal ratio, as in example C. This is termed "tridoshic Constitution." These folks are like chameleons, they really bring out different aspects of themselves depending on their energetic environs. For this reason, tri*dosha* predominant folks tend to be more affected by the energetics of their surroundings—the energy they take in drives which *dosha*(s) they get imbalanced in.

In a decade of practice, I haven't really seen anyone with a true single doshic predominance. About 70–80 percent of people present with a dual-doshic Constitution, and another 20–30 percent with a more tridoshic picture.

Notice all three of these examples are Pitta predominant. You likely have a good amount of Pitta too, as these folks are proactive about learning. Pitta predominants also usually have the Pitta traits of wanting to understand how things work, wanting to get better at a practice, wanting to spread knowledge, and the discipline and initiative to do yoga teacher training.

Pattern predominance

Not only are we made up of our parents' energy, but we are also imprinted with their patterns. Ancient sciences like the Vedas assert the passing on of energetic patterns across generations as an inherited cellular memory. Ancestral patterns are carried in maternal mitochondria, transcription regulating enzymes, and genetic code mutations which have been molded by the experience of the lives of our ancestors. We can look to the patterns of our parents and ancestors and better understand how to navigate our version of the same patterns, and how to support our children through their version of the same pattern.

Just as we discussed in the physical body, we can understand mental-emotional tendencies and patterns in the context of Constitution, and again, we can use awareness of these patterns to craft an approach to life that is going to give us the greatest balance. As in the physical body, our mental and emotional experience is one we can modulate. For example, if I know that I'm prone to over attachment, and staying, or holding on, I can bring in practices to help balance those Kaphic tendencies. I can implement supports to help me to release what's no longer serving me, and recenter my Kaphic attachment powers to things that serve me (e.g. attachment to my internal harmony, or to my ocean walks).

You are your parents, and that's okay.

It's helpful to understand that we are a mix of the patterns, so we will experience patterns that our parents did. We'll just experience them in different ways. Let me give an example to demonstrate. A client of mine had a mother who was never really able to prioritize the client's needs over her own. During the client's childhood, the mother repeatedly made choices which impacted my client in traumatic ways. The mother loved her daughter, but didn't have the capacity to mother her in a way that made my client feel safe and loved. Because of this, when the client became a mother herself, she chose to make mothering the most important task in her life. She prioritized the kids' needs over her own. Over time, she developed less tolerance to the kids, started smoking marijuana to help her relax around the kids, and kept putting off her own dreams in her creativity and work. My client had resources, a husband, and a nanny, but she felt she had to be the one to be there for everything for the kids. Even though she thought she was prioritizing the kids' needs, it was really her fear of being a bad mother that she was basing her choices on. My client's choices were a response to the internal guilt she felt about not meeting every one of the kids' needs herself. There was not a clear reason for her guilt—there was nothing to be guilty over as the kids' needs were all met and always had been. Her mother, on the other hand, likely did feel guilt. This was affirmed by how defensive she was with my client on this topic. What my client and I uncovered together is that she was engaging in the same emotional pattern of *guilt about mothering.* My client inherited the pattern of feeling like a guilty mother, and was mothering in response to that pattern. Our work then proceeded to help her parent from a place of meeting *both* the kids' and her own needs, and in shifting her patterned perspective that her meeting her needs would cause harm to her kids. We have all kinds of patterned ways of perceiving and responding to life, and we'll spend our lives learning these layers as yogis on the path of self-realization.

Common misperceptions

- *You cannot type yourself as one* dosha. At this point, you may already be able to understand that we cannot each simply be typed as Vata, Pitta, or Kapha. Vata, Pitta, and Kapha are together in every being, organ system, and cell. Make sure you have the word "predominant" when describing your Constitution.

- *Your goal is not to try to equal out your ratio.* Frequently, those new to Ayurveda ask if the goal of balance is to have equal amounts of Vata, Pitta, and Kapha. The answer is no. Your Constitution is *not* something we balance, or modulate. It's kind of like the vehicle of your life experience. The vehicle does have a big influence on how the drive feels, but the weather, road conditions, music, company in the car (akin to the major energetic inputs in your life) will be what really combine to determine the experience. What we are aiming to modify is not the vehicle, but the drive, which is our life experience. That's what we'll get into in the next chapter.

- *You are not powerless.* Another common misperception of Constitution is the idea that if we have a set energetic ratio, we cannot change who we are. This becomes especially relevant when we consider inherited diseases. If we consistently change our life experience, or health experience, it *will* change who we are to some degree. We can affect the expression of the genetic disease pattern.

  While our Constitution (*prakruti*) reveals our set point, and thus our innate tendencies, our life experience is a continuing input of energy. We can make shifts in our Constitution with long-term or significant energy inputs (e.g. pregnancy, 40 years of farming, 20 years of regular international work travel, 15 years of raw food diet, 10 years of an abusive relationship). Going back to the vehicle analogy, what we put the vehicle through does affect the vehicle over time. In other words, the vehicle starts to incorporate the experience too.

- *We're not here to to fix your Constitution.* The main purpose of assessing your Constitution is to understand your core tendencies, habits, and patterns. Then, we accept these defaults. We accept that this is how we were made in this lifetime, and we love ourselves as we are. You can see how Ayurveda is inherently a self-loving way of life. Once you have a clear sense of your patterns, you can customize ways to support your wellbeing.

Personally, I can appreciate the wealth of information my Constitution may give me about my tendencies, but that's not what I *most* appreciate. The truth is if you engage in any regular practice of building awareness of your patterns/habits/tendencies, you'll get a good sense of them without a Constitution analysis. What I most appreciate about my Constitution is the opportunity to build compassion for my natural ways of operating, and learn how to best support myself.

I don't need to judge myself for having a short temper. I can simply understand that it's an artifact of my Pitta predominant nature—this is how I was put together. I can honor that *same* Pitta predominance that allows me ease in learning, teaching, and spreading information.

Seeing how your challenges are also gifts is an amazing practice for those of us with a natural tendency to be hard on ourselves (ahem, all of us Pitta predominants).

I accept the short temper, and learn to support myself better for that trait. For example, now I do Pitta reducing breathing when I feel my temper flaring, or tell my family that I need to go chill because I'm about to blow. Because I accept this about myself, and am working with it, my family does too. They don't take it personally when I flare, and give me the space to go cool off. When we acknowledge and work with who we are, the people in our lives are more likely to do so.

Assessing Constitutions

The best way to assess your Constitution is by physical exam which relies heavily on pulse and body features, such as tongue, nail, palm, facial line, and iris readings. Practitioners and doctors of Ayurveda are trained to see the qualities of VPK in these traits.

The next best way, perhaps more accurate at times, is via Vedic astrology. Vedic astrology is a beautifully complex energetic mapping system itself, and much more than the *prakruti*, or Constitution, can be mapped. Adept Vedic astrologers can map when you will have specific ailments in specific parts of your body. There are people who practice both Vedic Astrology and Ayurveda, as both are practices of mapping energetic patterns.

Ayurvedic Constitution questionnaires are ubiquitous, and can be helpful in figuring out your personal ratio, or Constitution. The idea behind surveys is to offer a glimpse into your nature when you don't have an Ayurvedic practitioner around. Surveys are easy, and their simplicity also renders them limited. Appendix 2 is a *Constitution Survey* and it's available as a download.[1] My main purpose in providing this is for you to see how limited they are in their accuracy and application.

Limitations of a Constitution-centered approach

In my opinion, the Constitution is less important than the Current State of energetics when we consider how to balance ourselves. Approaching

---

1   www.ayurvedabysiva.com/worksheets

healing has to be tailored to where you are today. In other words, directions to any destination are relative to the starting place.

Every Ayurvedic website or book offers a Constitutional survey. Then they offer balancing suggestions based on Constitution. This Constitution-centered approach is limited in its effectiveness because it fails to take into account energetics of your life journey. If I'm Pitta predominant, but have decades of high Vata imbalance, trying to balance Pitta wouldn't serve me well and it would likely aggravate my Vata imbalance. This is why I don't subscribe to the type-yourself-and-live-this-way approach. This labeling mentality is a part of modern culture, from labeling what kind of yoga you practice, to what your love language is, to eating for your blood type.

We are are incorporating the energy of our lives into our very cells and neural circuits. With this in mind, we can appreciate how very unique we each are. No one can have the exact same energy exposure throughout life as someone else, even twins. It makes so much sense to tailor a healing approach, or lifestyle approach based on our unique nature *and* life experience, and this is my approach to Ayurveda.

Constitutions and karmic lessons

By the time we reach our 20s, we know our core patterns. You know how your sleep, digestion, and emotions trend, and what aggravates and soothes those trends. We're not here to solve the trends or baseline patterns. We can't. If I was made with a strong tendency towards inflammation, I'm not going to cure that. Instead, I'm going to learn to work with it and tailor my lifestyle to balance inflammation.

In Vedic thought, we all have certain karmic patterns in this lifetime. Our Constitutional patterns are the set up for those karmic lessons. Our experience of parents, our childhoods, our early imprints—these are our *samskaras*. How you experience your early years—how you imprint—is like your inherited blueprint on how to receive and respond to life. Our Constitutions play a big role in how we originally receive and respond to life. As we learn our karmic lessons, we learn to navigate our old imprinted patterns and cultivate new ones.

Learning to work with your nature is learning to accept yourself.

Learning to love and work with who you are, as you are, *is the new pattern*. In learning how to respond to life differently, in the new pattern, we fulfil our karmic lessons. This doesn't mean they go away forever, but they appear less frequently, and with less intensity.

For example, if I have a Pitta predominance and a core pattern to be intense, that intensity will be my default. I likely learned this way of intensity from my family, or as a reaction to my family. Most people are too distracted in modern life to be present with how they are experiencing life, and with how they want to receive and respond to life. If I'm able to become aware, over time, I'll see the suffering caused by my intensity, for me and for my loved ones. I'll want to change the default and experience a new pattern—one that doesn't feel intense.

In growing my awareness and shifting my responses, I fulfill my karmic lesson. In my new pattern, I value down time, play, and supporting myself to not feel so intense. The new experience, being able to experience life without much intensity, is the prize for, and proof of, my micro-evolution.

The tendency to be intense, to feel intense, is with me for life—it's just that I've trained myself to feel otherwise. Imagine a pose where there is a certain tendency you've noticed and chosen to work on— let's say not tightening your face muscles in *Tadasana*. You may still do that on occasion, even after years, but maybe less so. Maybe you catch it faster and train yourself to relax your facial muscles in many intense poses. What I'm aiming to change is the *frequency, severity, duration,* and negative consequences of my core patterns/imprint/Constitutional patterns *samskaras*. When I grow my awareness and apply that to my life choices, *that is spiritual growth.*

So, your family and childhood imprint, messes you up in *exactly the right way* for you to seek to shift; to learn what you need to in this life for your unique spiritual growth plan. We're not here to blame them for our ways. We had to experience the pain of our ways to birth the desire for the new pattern. All new patterns are achievable. You may regress into old patterns when in old energetics, like family dynamics. The Vedic teacher Ram Das acknowledged this old pattern triggering when he quipped, "If you think you are enlightened, go spend a week with your family."

The speed at which you shift into a new pattern will simply depend on how much resistance you have inside you to stay as you are. As animals, it's instinctive to stick to perspectives and behaviors of those who have survived. Behavior patterns are encoded in DNA for this reason. The idea is to copy whatever the animals before you did to survive and make it to procreation and imprinting young ones. It's the norm to stick with what you know. We're evolved enough to choose to imprint after those who are thriving in life, not just surviving.

Your core patterns will remain. It's your awareness that changes.

Summary

- Constitution is your ratio of Vata, Pitta, and Kapha.

- Constitution determines your

  - physical structure

  - major personality traits

  - core vulnerabilities and strengths.

- Constitution doesn't take into account life experience.

You can now get a sense of your Constitution. Simply take a look at your core features and patterns, and you'll start to see the *doshas* in your nature. Constitution is helpful for self acceptance and long-term prevention, but it's actually not where I focus for balancing. That's our Current State, which we'll cover next!

Use the *Constitution Survey* (Appendix 2) to assess yourself. Please read the directions as I overview a lot of common questions that come up with filling out this survey. Once you've completed the survey, you should be able to complete these summary sentences:

I have a *(single, dual, or tri)* doshic
predominance in my Constitution.

My Constitution is predominantly (V, P, K or some combination).

We're not trying to change you. We're just getting to know you on another level.

Next, we'll start tapping into what your body and mind are telling us about your Current State.

Chapter 5

YOUR CURRENT STATE

Importance of Current State and How to Assess Imbalances

Learning objectives

- Understand what Current State is, and what factors play into your Current State.

- Be able to see how Current State determines healing choices.

- Understand how your body and mind are revealing their energetic patterns.

- Get a sense of your own Current State.

What is Current State?

In Ayurveda, we acknowledge that where you are today may be quite a different energetic ratio than what you were created with. You are a big energy ball that interacts with the energy surrounding you, and that has incorporated the energy from your life experience since you were born. The Sanskrit term for "where you are at," or Current State, as I like to call it, is *vikruti*—Current State as the result of your Constitution interfacing with your life experiences.

Because Current State is in constant flux, ratio is not a useful parameter with Current State the way it is in Constitutions. The reason I want to know my Current State is to know how to approach feeling better. So, let's define Current State as our *current levels of imbalance*. If we know which imbalances we have, and which ones are the greatest, we can address them more directly and strategically. To feel good as soon as possible, I'll go for addressing the biggest imbalances, the ones causing me the most pain, first.

We discussed in the last chapter how our Constitutional predominance gives us certain imbalance tendencies. Because I have a lot of Pitta qualities, I don't need too much more before I feel like I have more Pitta qualities than I feel good with. As soon as I have what feels like too much Pitta, I'll start to show signs of excessive Pitta in my mind and tissues.

What determines Current State?

We are are incorporating the energy of our lives into our very cells and neural circuits. With this in mind, we can again appreciate how very unique your Current State is. No one can have the exact same energy exposure throughout life as anyone else, not even identical twins.

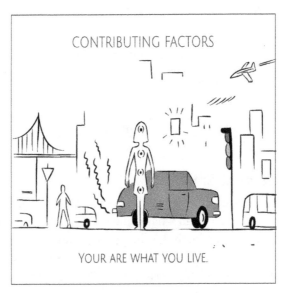

Figure 5.1 *You are what you live*

Every experience in life is an input of energy. Let me repeat that for dramatic emphasis: *Every* experience in life is an energetic input. Your commute, your sleep, your conversations, your food, your loved ones— you are taking it all in, and becoming it, literally.

If you live in a very dry climate, you'll take in the quality of dryness, and eventually, your body tissues will become more dry. Your speech and your perspectives may also reflect greater quality of dryness. Tropical island dwellers maintain more supple tissues because of their more supple surroundings, and their speech may be more fluid and deep pitched, like the water that surrounds them. Over the course of generations, body structures become more heavy and wide because of the greater qualities of water and earth in tropical islands.

These are simply examples of how we take in the qualities of our physical climate. Now, imagine what qualities you are taking in your life's emotional climates. When I first realized this, I thought, "Oh no!" (and that's normal). There's little value to judging your life so far and being hard on yourself—internal conflict is not good for your health. Let's agree, instead, to use this awareness, to be inspired by it, and actively cultivate the energetics of our life experiences to match what we need!

The people in our lives are also a big energetic input, as are our relationships with them. Not only do I take in the energy of my partner, but also the energy of our co-created relationship. So I can have a Pitta predominant partner, and a very easy stable nurturing (Kapha) predominant relationship energetic. In this example, I'd be taking in both the Pitta of my partner, and the Kapha of our relationship.

It's worth paying attention to how you feel around different people, and this is a variable phenomenon. With the same person, we can feel challenged or supported. Meditation, or the *sthira*, that we get from our yoga practice helps us *cope* with the energetics. However, it doesn't make us aware of the energetic input and how it affects our bodies and hearts.

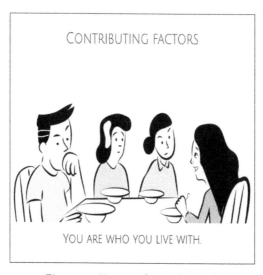

Figure 5.2 *You are who you live with*

We are not here to blame others for our Current State, but rather to understand some of how we got here, to better guide us in moving towards *where we want to be*. We can use Ayurveda as a way to understand what our needs are from our interactions with people as well. If I know where I am energetically, and what kinds of energy an interaction tends to bring, it's easy to see whether that is a fit for me that day. For example, I may choose to not take a call from my super-Pitta intense friend on a day when I'm feeling like I need easy, sweet, and light energetics.

This means that you selectively choose your interactions with people the way you do your food— based on the energy you're taking in. *Is salad a good fit for me today? Is spending time with Mom a good fit for me today?* It's all just energy, and I can choose based on what feels best that day.

You may find that those around you have similar energetic patterns (e.g. self-deprecating humor, healthy eating habits, workaholism), and it's common for us to attract people who have similar Current State energetics in our lives. For example, if I have a lot of Pitta, it's likely my family does too. I naturally gravitate towards people that have high Pitta qualities because it's familiar. Perhaps I choose people that are ambitious, research and analyze, and have an competitive edge. I respect these qualities in them, because I have them myself. However, spending time with them could result in cerebral, intense, sometimes defensive interactions that bring in more Pitta. I'm not saying that you cannot spend time with people that have similar qualities to you. I'm asserting that we can be aware of what energy we take in from the people in our lives, and adjust it according to what we need *that day*.

Most humans have many many sides to themselves, and our different faces come out with different people or situations. Once you understand this, you aim to interact with the person in a way that matches your goal of being well and happy. Our focus here is not on their behavior, but rather our response. The change in any relationship dynamic starts with you (and that's another book!)

Oftentimes, as we shift the energetics of our lives, we will shift the people that are the main players in our lives, or the dynamics of the main relationships. In other words, as you start to pay attention to how you feel after spending time with people—what energetics you take in from them—you may want to spend less time with them. Many people can see how the energetics of relationship dynamics are playing into their imbalances once they begin paying attention. This is natural, and common. So be forewarned that growing your awareness can lead to having to make some tough choices about the people in your life.

Where are the imbalances coming from?

If you have signs and symptoms of a *dosha* in your body or mind, you must have brought in that *dosha* through your recent life experiences. I just presented climate and people as two examples of major energetic inputs. Our energetic inputs are much more than that—we're taking it all in. It would be overwhelming to constantly categorize the energy of all we experience in life. That's not worth the effort or time, because we're more concerned with the major sources of *doshas* we are imbalanced in. For our example of a Pitta predominant woman with Vata imbalance, we just want to identify the *major sources* of Vata for her at present. We want to look at where the excess *dosha* is coming in from, so we can target the interventions.

We began looking at which *doshas* are coming into your life in the *VPK in My Life Worksheet* (Appendix 1, also available as a PDF download).[1] We considered the *doshas* coming in from your work, routine, food, and closest relationship. These are *big* energetic inputs. A weekend yoga intensive workshop, for example, may have a lot of V and P that you take in, but it's just for that weekend. Once you are regularly fine tuning the approach to your life based on what is happening that day, or week, you would consider that and bring in balancing adjustments to counterbalance the energy of the workshop. However, for our purposes now, we want to see the energetics of the *most significant* energetic inputs and get a big-picture understanding of what you are bringing in energetically. Even if you don't have any health concerns, it's helpful to see the major energetics of your life, as they will determine your imbalances.

Shifting the focus from Constitution to Current State

Constitution-based advice, which you'll find in a lot of Ayurveda online, focuses on recommendations that are based on your most predominant *dosha*, not on your most prominent imbalances *today*. Our Current State, where we are energetically at this moment, is more relevant to current ailments than our Constitution.

---

1   www.ayurvedabysiva.com/worksheets

In the discussion about Constitutions, I mentioned that we are more likely to go out of balance in the *doshas* that are predominant in our Constitution. You can use this awareness of your predominances to set up a more balancing lifestyle over the *long term*. However, most of us are blessed to just be able to feel well in the now, and strategizing a lifelong health plan based on tendencies is a bit idealistic. This is why I present Ayurveda as a practice of reflecting on "*Where am I at? What do I need?*"—it's self inquiry and response to your Current State. Once you get good at sensing where you are energetically and making balancing choices, then you can consider long-term lifestyle choices based on your long-term patterns.

Because your Current State reflects your Constitution, if we focus on Current State, we're inherently attending to Constitutional tendencies. In other words, "Where am I at?" *includes* consideration of how you were made. Someone with a Pitta predominance is likely to show Pitta often in their current imbalances. If any *dosha* needs balancing, it will show itself in our bodies and minds, and we respond accordingly. In a lifestyle of attentively responding to where I'm at and what I need *in the present*, a sophisticated analysis of how I was made becomes irrelevant.

Let's consider a Pitta predominant person with mostly Vata symptoms, after having gone through high Vata life experience. Her healing would start by addressing her Vata imbalances, because that's where her symptoms and suffering are. Of course, we can fine tune our approach with awareness of Constitutional tendencies. So, in this case, we'd go for balancing her Vata symptoms, while being mindful of not bringing in too much qualities of Pitta.

If the majority of her symptoms are Vata; if Vata symptoms span the greatest number of tissues or systems; if Vata symptoms have been around the longest, or become chronic; or if Vata symptoms cause her greatest suffering, I'm going to recommend a Vata balancing lifestyle. When I'm attending to what her body is telling us now, it really doesn't matter what her Constitution is.

Healing starts in the now.

I'll go into balancing more in the next chapter. For now, the key point is that our healing approach begins with a focus on Current State. Irrespective of your Constitution, your Current State is the *most* important determinant of your healing approach, because *where you are at* now is where your healing must begin.

How do I know if I have an imbalance?

Our Current State can be assessed through our *present* state of emotions and physical condition. If everything is functioning perfectly and I feel wonderful, that's when I'm free of imbalance. I haven't met anyone yet in modern urban life that is free of any sign of imbalance. Part of the beauty, and power, of Ayurveda is that you can notice the first signs of imbalance, and that's way before you have a full blown diagnosis.

If I'm experiencing symptoms, then I have imbalances. If the quality of a *dosha* is associated with a symptom, that *dosha* must be out of balance in that part of the body. By examining how our tissues feel, and their functions, we identify qualities (e.g. hot, cold, dry, painful, swollen, heavy). From the qualities, we identify which *doshas* are involved, or "imbalanced," and where. If I have symptoms with qualities of Vata in my mind-state (e.g. scattered, restless), then I have Vata imbalance in my mind and nervous system. If I have symptoms with qualities of Pitta in my digestion (e.g. heat, inflammation), I have Pitta imbalance in my digestive system. If I have symptoms with qualities of Kapha in my uterus or prostate (e.g. accumulating growth as in fibroids or enlarged prostate), then I have Kapha imbalance in my reproductive system. The *doshas* that are involved in the *most parts of you* are the ones with the most imbalance in.

Assessing your Current State

Our Current State can be assessed through the qualities of our present state of emotions and physical tissues. We'll look at solving the imbalances in the next chapter. Here, we're more focused on *sensing the imbalances* and the *doshas* involved.

As described above, we check in with the information our various tissue systems are giving us—the qualities of their physical structure and functions will tell us which *doshas* are at play. Let's practice a bit. In the chart below, I've listed out sample symptoms in a few different parts of the body. For each symptom, I've associated a core quality, and the *dosha* revealed by that symptom-quality.

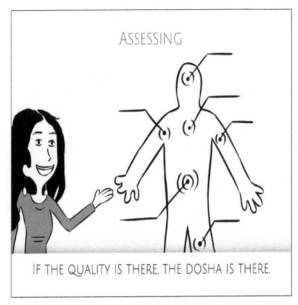

Figure 5.3 *Qualities reveal* doshas *in the body and mind*

Chart 5.1 Symptoms, qualities and *doshas* in various tissues

Tissue, organ or function	Symptoms—qualities	*Dosha*
Emotional body	anxious—unknown restless—unsettled racing thoughts—movement	V
Digestion	hyperacidity—heat inflammation—heat ulceration—spreading	P
Skin	dry—dry discolored—irregular	V
Sinuses membranes	congested—blocked mucous—slimy	K

It will take some time for you to pick up the language of your body and emotions. Until then, I've created a reference tool elucidating the *doshas* in the most common symptoms: *Signs of Imbalance Chart* (Appendix 3). This will help you to begin to understand what your tissues are saying. We'll use this tool to take a look at your Current State at the end of this chapter. In other words, we're going to start decoding what our bodies and emotions are telling us. Our tissues are in constant communication with us. It's just that we haven't been taught their language, *or to listen.*

We are constantly feeling emotions, but remain unaware that are feelings are how our emotional bodies are communicating with our minds. We have little understanding of what the emotions are telling us, and how to respond—this is what we'll go over in Chapter 9. Similarly, I hope to decode what your digestive system is communicating in Chapter 8. As with any language, the more time you spend with it, the more skilled and aware of subtleties you become.

Your perspective matters

Because this entails observation of you, how you feel is incredibly relevant. Ultimately, you are the best assessor of yourself (and maybe that's in progress). Most of us have a feeling that things just aren't quite feeling right in our bodies, or our emotional bodies, and that's usually the first sign of imbalance.

In the beginning, people feel like they need a practitioner to assess their imbalances. While practitioners can reveal things to us about ourselves, the truth is that no one can better sense what the qualitative feel of your body and emotions than you. So really, the best practitioners, in my opinion, are teaching you how to better sense yourself.

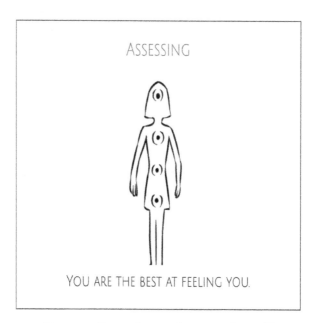

Figure 5.4 *You can be a good assessor of yourself*

Let's say a man had inflamed arthritis in his hands, which worsened after use, and felt hot. These are all Pitta qualities that suggest this arthritis experience is a sign of Pitta imbalance. If his arthritis presented with no inflammation, stiffness and cracking-popping in the joints, worse in the morning and better after moving around, and worse in cold weather, the qualities of his arthritis—stiff, dry, cold, rigid—are all qualities of Vata imbalance.

In the example above, no one but the man himself could reveal the qualities of his arthritis. With practice, and maybe a bit of guidance and validation from a practitioner, you can become adept at sensing which *doshas* are out of balance in your various parts.

Sensing vs. analyzing

Your five senses are the perfect starting place to begin sensing energy. The more you trust your senses, the more you will trust yourself, and the easier decision making will become.

Part of what makes Ayurveda so universal is that anyone with sense organs can sense energy. However, in today's modern urban setting, we would rather analyze. In other words, we are more comfortable trusting our brains to apply a learned science, than trusting our ability to feel or sense. It's not uncommon for me to have to ask how someone feels about a situation a few times before I actually get them to use feeling words, and not simply express what they *think*.

So, if learning this science of Ayurveda and applying the "rules" is more comfortable than feeling it for you, you are not alone. And in reality, there is a lot of learning in the beginning of these new concepts. I'll encourage you to start this journey as a more academic one, and eventually develop it into a more intuitive one.

For example, I can have you memorize a list of symptoms as signs of Vata imbalance in the digestive tract. Then when you note a symptom, your brain will say, "ah, that's Vata excess in your digestive system." Eventually, you will feel dryness in your stool, and know that Vata is present because you've associated the *feeling* of dryness with Vata.

Sensing the *doshas* is a more powerful and thorough approach than memorizing lists. *What if a symptom is not on the list? What if it feels like a combination of two different symptoms?* The qualities you sense will reveal exactly which *dosha*(s) need to be balanced irrespective of a list.

A great example of this is the Ayurvedic food chart. Let's say I have a banana, which is traditionally listed as a Kapha food due to its sweet, slimy, dense, and nutritive qualities. Now, let's say this was an unripe banana. As I ate it, I felt dryness in my mouth, bitterness and it felt more rigid than soft. This unripe banana had a lot of Vata qualities, and would be a Vata input based on my experience, which I may erroneously think of as a Kapha input based on the chart and my brain. Similarly, a super sweet and juicy giant heirloom tomato could be very Kaphic, while all tomatoes are categorized as Pitta, as they are traditionally tart and acidic.

We can't chart every possibility, so depending more and more on your senses is how you slowly build trust to allow your awareness of the *doshas* to become a natural thing. In the beginning, it will seem like you have to think a lot to decide how to balance; in time, decision making becomes more effortless.

Healing choices based on Current State

Getting in tune with your patterns may take some practice. Before Ayurveda, I didn't really look at my poop regularly, or know if my bowel movements were optimal. It was a sign of how unplugged I was with my bodily patterns, and this is common in modern urban lifestyle. Oftentimes this is because we are overstimulated, and/or caught up in our worries, and/or escaping our reality with TV, Facebook, etc.

Because we all have imbalances all the time, occurring and resolving, or occurring and progressing, your Current State will change. Oftentimes there are patterns.

Ayurveda helps you choose what is best for you in any given moment. I emphasize "given moment" because we are dynamic beings with ever changing needs and experiences. What is best for me in the summer may be different than in the winter. I will have different needs in diet, herbs, routine, etc. when I have a cold, when I'm premenstrual, when I'm stressed out, postpartum, post-andropause, or traveling, for example.

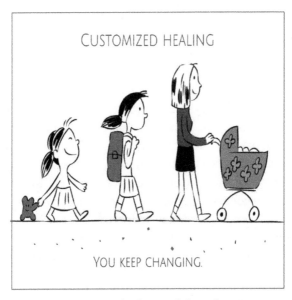

Figure 5.5 *Your healing needs keep changing*

We look at signs of imbalance to assess *what is needed* to best balance the Current State. In other words, Current State awareness is what will guide our decision making. On a day when I know my body is communicating a lot of qualities of Pitta, I'm going to make choices to decrease my Pitta intake—perhaps in my food, my work, my exercise. And I'm going to make choices to bring in balancing for Pitta as well, which is what we'll cover in the next chapter.

We're never going to solve it all. Our aim is to *be in touch with ourselves*, and choose according to this increased awareness of our Current State.

Change isn't always easy or fast

When you are learning to really pay attention, you will become more sensitive and more aware. This means *you are about to change*. Time and time again, I witness people on their Ayurvedic journey no longer enjoying the company of some people, or foods, or habits. And it can mean that the awareness of how your life is affecting you leads you to change your job or relationships. With this increased awareness, you may shift in what you seek in food, relationships, work, etc.

Because you are listening more, and more connected to yourself, you will also become a bit more intuitive. These are all good things, but can sometimes be challenging parts of growing and healing. On the flipside of every challenge is the growth or healing opportunity—that's where we want to focus.

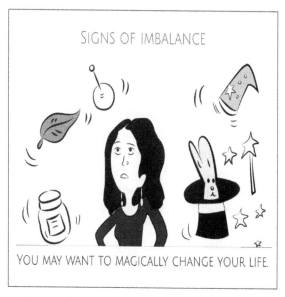

Figure 5.6 *Once you become aware, you may wish you had a magic wand*

Summary

- Current State looks at your levels of imbalance.
- Current State is a direct reflection of life energetics.
- Your body and feelings are (trying) to talk to you.
- Categorize imbalances by qualities.
- Current State determines healing approach.
- Increased awareness of your life energetics can be challenging.

Now, let's get a sense of your imbalances. Use the *Signs of Imbalance Chart* (Appendix 3) to take inventory of your body and emotions, and this will reveal your Current State. Summarize the findings for your physical body and your psychospiritual body as follows:

I have mostly signs of *(V, P, K or some combination)* imbalance in my mind and emotions.

I have mostly signs of (V, P, K or some combination) imbalance in my body.

The *Signs of Imbalance Chart* (Appendix 3) is a great place to start listening to what your body and your emotions are revealing to you about your energetic state. My intention with this chart is to offer a simple tool to help get you started. Let's acknowledge the limitations of this tool: my words may not be the way you describe what you feel; and the list of qualities and symptoms is not all-inclusive. For this reason, I've provided a blank *Current State Survey* (Appendix 4). You can fill out this chart utilizing your own descriptions of what you're feeling, and it's open to everything you're feeling.

I'd recommend starting with the *Signs of Imbalance Chart*, and continuing to use this until you're comfortable sensing VPK signs, or describing what you feel. At this point, move onto using the *Current State Survey*. In the *Current State Survey*, you'll notice some additional reflections. By considering which *doshas* have the most signs of imbalance, the longest standing, and cause us the greatest bother, we are getting clear on priorities for making balancing choices. This clarity will serve us in the next chapter when we explore this process of finding balance.

Chapter 6

BALANCING

Learning objectives

- Be able to define imbalance.

- Review common misperceptions about imbalances and balancing.

- Understand how to assess for a balancing.

- Get a sense of the major balancing approaches in Ayurveda.

In the previous chapter, I emphasized that Current State determines what you will choose as balancing tools or choices. Your Constitution, and what's going on in your life, will help us fine tune those choices. In this chapter, I'll define imbalance in Ayurveda, and then guide you through balancing approaches. We'll use your *Signs of Imbalance Chart* findings to explore where to start making some balancing shifts in your own life.

Our learning objectives are to be able to define imbalance, understand how it occurs, and have a beginning sense about what to do to feel better.

What is imbalance?

Let's start by defining imbalance. In Ayurveda, imbalance is always viewed as a state of *excess*. Every symptom is described as too much of a certain energy. Even if we are feeling depleted, or "low in energy," Ayurveda would describe this as a state of excess depletion. Instead of saying I didn't have enough heat, I would say I have excessive cold. For any quality that you are feeling deficient in, we'd say you have *too much of its opposite.* This is brilliant because it really helps to keep things simple. Whatever is showing up as too much is what we address. That's it.

Recall that our tissues are reflecting what we are taking *in*, in life. We're taking in the energy of our lives and making ourselves up of it. So, when considering what is being felt by those tissues, we are looking at what's coming in excessively. If I have signs of Vata in my tissues, then that's my body telling me that I have *too much* Vata coming into those tissues. I could call this "Vata imbalance" or "Vata excess." With the above example of feeling cold, I could say I have a "Vata imbalance" in my circulatory system, or too much Vata in my blood, and these are all synonymous.

Returning to the big-picture definitions I gave of VPK in Chapter 3, we can get a big-picture understanding of VPK imbalances. Since V is an unpredictable, degenerative energy, it makes sense that V imbalances all involve *degeneration, depletion, or irregularity.* As P is a spreading, heating energy, we can understand that P imbalances involve *inflammation and infection.* With K energy's growing heavy nature, it follows that K imbalances are due to *accumulation, stagnation, and stuckness.* You may have noticed this perspective of VPK imbalance at the top of the *Signs of Imbalance Chart.* This big picture view may make it easier to understand what kinds of imbalance you are experiencing, and why.

I have never met a situation where no balancing is needed. To me, the idea of being free of any symptoms is hypothetical. Just like there is no perfect yoga practice—it's always shifting to feel slightly better that day.

Imbalance = too much *dosha*(s) coming in through life

No symptoms = *doshas* are balanced in life = unlikely

Symptoms present = your tissues saying, "Enough is enough"

When your tissues are showing signs and symptoms of the *doshas*, they're telling you "I've had enough." Because we're not raised to listen to these signs from the body, or to understand the language of the body, we usually ignore the signs, and continue making imbalancing choices.

Before even hearing about Ayurveda, I'm sure there has been a time where you *listened to your body.* Maybe you took a sick day to rest in bed, or cancelled plans to ground yourself—even something as simple as eating when hungry, or drinking when thirsty counts. I promise you that *every time* you did this, your body gave you a "thumbs up" in the most profound way—*feeling good.*

Simply because you're paying attention, you're going to start "hearing" your tissues in a deeper way. This increased connection with your inner guidance system translates into less internal conflict and anxiety, more confidence, more clarity, stronger intuition, and greater health.

Common misperceptions about imbalances

There are a lot of opinions out there on what balance is and how to achieve it. Perhaps the best way to convey some of the subtleties of balancing is to address common misperceptions on Ayurveda and imbalance.

You can have more than one imbalance, and most do

Imbalance result from the choices we're making in life, when those choices expose us to too much of VPK. Because we're always taking in a blend of energetics, we often have imbalances in multiple *doshas*. It's common to have more than one *dosha* out of balance in your Current State. From what I'm seeing, most people over the age of 20, in modern urban settings, have imbalance in all three *doshas* concurrently. Urban lifestyles are further removed from nature's rhythms and have more Vata (screentime, processed food, transitions) and are thus more imbalancing, even if you have your kids in a great private school, and do yoga everyday, and eat organic. Imbalances are happening earlier and earlier, as disconnection with our emotional bodies and body signals is happening earlier.

Imbalance is usually caused by more than one factor

The Western approach to pathogenesis is quite linear: this caused that. So, Western thinking commonly follows this approach: *"I have bad gas because I'm gluten intolerant."* In the more circular Eastern approach, we view everything as related and summative. The bad gas would be understood in the greater context of how it came about—lots of Vata piling up in the digestive system after years of a Vata lifestyle, and lots of Vata food, resulting in weak digestion that cannot handle heavy foods, like gluten.

The Eastern approach is more powerful because the bigger picture and the higher number of factors involved provide more ways to shift the situation and heal. When I use the linear single-factor approach, I can only remove gluten from the diet. The person will likely remain with Vata imbalance in the digestive system, and not understand why removing the gluten didn't solve all their digestive symptoms.

With the broader multi-factor approach, I will likely decrease gluten for some time to not stress out the digestive system while I rehabilitate it. The longer term goal would be to decrease the Vata coming into the digestive system by decreasing Vata in the foods and the lifestyle. This means I'm rejuvenating the weakened part of the body, increasing awareness of the sources of the imbalance, and making choices to shift the energetics towards my goal of balancing Vata. Incidentally, I've seen many people improve their ability to digest heavy foods, which used to trigger them, using this more comprehensive approach.

There is no magic state of balance

I'm realizing that balance is not something we can just achieve. Life keeps bringing inputs of energetics, and we continuously need to shift to respond and find again what feels like homeostasis. The body is in a constant state of flux, responding to external inputs to maintain internal balance, and so is our emotional body. We'll have happy days and days that feel good in our bodies, but we cannot expect to not be affected by our lifestyles and stress.

Our goal is not to achieve an idealized balance state. Rather, we're here to acknowledge where we are at, and what we need to feel good in that particular time-space reality.

Imbalances signal us when we need to shift the energetics of our lives. We can honor them as messengers that go away once we've made the balancing shifts. As we go into assessing, it may be helpful to remember this is just a practice of self-inquiry, and increasing our awareness and acceptance.

Assessing imbalances

The main part of assessing imbalances is looking at Current State, or symptoms, as we did in the last chapter. There are some additional assessment considerations that can help us fine tune our approach. We can get a better sense of *what you need*, and *where to start*, by understanding the degree, duration, depth, and sources of your imbalances.

We explored the presence and degree of imbalance in the *Signs of Imbalance Chart* and the *Current State Survey* (Chapter 5, Appendices 3 and 4). After completing these exercises you should know if you have multiple imbalances and which ones are the greatest. To review, the *doshas* you have the most symptoms of are the ones in which you have the greatest degree of imbalance. When we have signs of imbalance in all three *doshas*, it's helpful to consider the degree of the imbalance. The *dosha* with the greatest amount, or degree, of imbalance will be the one we want to address foremost.

My body will give me the first signs that there is too much VPK by showing me the qualities and symptoms in my tissues and emotions. If I *continue* to bring in the same energetics from all my inputs, I'm going to further the imbalance. In other words, I'm continuing to increase what is already feeling like too much. This will show by increased duration, frequency, or severity of the symptoms—which I like to view as increased *depth* of imbalance.

Usually, imbalances that have been around for a long time have more depth, or severity. I often see people whose Vata signs reflect the greatest degree of imbalance, have been around the longest, and are in the most tissue systems. It's common to have the most and the longest-standing signs in the same *dosha*. However, it doesn't have to be this way. I could, for example, have a woman who has had Vata symptoms around the longest, but is post-menopausal, and with mostly Pitta signs currently. Anything is possible, and all must be considered on an individual basis.

We want to know which imbalance is the greatest degree, duration, or depth, because this helps us prioritize which imbalance to address first.

Focus on the big problem first.

Next, we want to consider the sources of these energetics. We started this practice with the *VPK in My Life Worksheet* (Appendix 1). It's not always a clean cut story. We can bring in *doshas* in any combo across any area of life, and it's changing. We focus on the now and on building awareness.

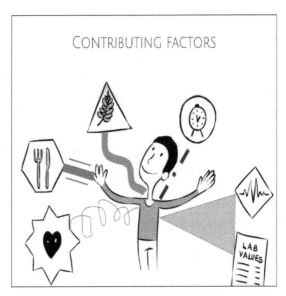

Figure 6.1 *All life energetics contribute to Current State*

Let's say a man has imbalances in V, P, and K. His *Current State Survey* reveals that V is most imbalanced and P is not far behind. His V symptoms cause him the most suffering, and have been around the longest. The V symptoms span non-physical and physical, and are the most prominent in his body. The P symptoms are more so in his mind and emotions. When we look at the sources of his imbalances, he has too much V coming in from his food, his routine, his major relationship, and his age. Simultaneously, he's bringing in too much P from work and exercise. Concurrently, he has too much K coming in with his diet (e.g. soothing with carbs).

There's no exact science on how to approach this balancing path—it's an art. But having all the above information allows us to sense that V is really the focus of his balancing efforts. And we're going to target V decreasing efforts in the areas of life that are bringing in the most V.

To get to the point of having regular symptoms, it's likely that imbalance will have built up across a few areas of life, over time—in his case the Vata imbalance from too much V in diet, routine, relationships, and age. This is why looking for *at least three sources* of whichever *dosha* is imbalanced is a great practice. Sometimes, there is an obvious singular cause for something, like food poisoning and digestive symptoms. However, even in these cases, we can likely find other contributing factors, such as poor sleep and high stress leading to immune depletion that contributed to the foodborne infection happening more easily. In the broader multi-factorial approach of Ayurveda, having more sources for the imbalance gives us more targets for healing interventions.

Secondary imbalances

Thus far, we've only discussed primary imbalances—ones that come in obviously, and directly from VPK excess. When an imbalance has been around for long enough, oftentimes the body tries to heal itself. The body's response can lead to a secondary imbalance—one that is in response to a primary imbalance.

The majority of ailments in the body are degenerative, malfunctioning, infective or inflammatory. In other words, 90 percent of what can go wrong with the body involves Vata and Pitta in excess. When we don't address our imbalances for a certain amount of time, the body does what it can to protect itself. Kapha is a protective energy, so it makes sense that a lot of the body's healing responses are to accumulate Kapha.

It's common to mount a secondary Kapha imbalance in response to Vata and Pitta imbalances we've had for a while. In the chart below, I've listed some of the common secondary accumulations of Kapha, in response to long-standing Vata and Pitta in these tissues. Even in the emotional body, long-standing Vata and Pitta issues/imbalances/excuses, such as anxiety and pressure to solve, can result in a secondary Kaphic depression. If you've had signs of Vata and Pitta *preceding* your Kapha symptoms in any part of your body, there's a good chance that it's a secondary Kapha imbalance.

Chart 6.1 Longstanding imbalances can lead to secondary imbalances

Primary imbalance	Secondary imbalance
dry or inflamed sinus membranes	mucous
depleted or inflamed reproductive tissues	polyps, fibroids, ovarian cysts, enlarged prostates
dry, cracked skin	callous
fatigued thyroid	goiter, weight gain
dry, cracked arteries	cholesterol plaques
dry, inflamed eyes	cataracts

People can have Kaphic symptoms from primary Kapha imbalance too. In other words, they are *not* always a response to longstanding Vata and/or Pitta. This would happen if they have a lot of Kapha in their Constitution *and* their lives. I find, however, in modern urban living, that this is rare, because Kapha qualities—like stable, still, nurturing, safe, and supported—are rarer in our lives.

Further, you can have Kapha imbalances that are part primary and part secondary. In other words, too much Kapha coming in directly from some areas of life (primary), and some Kapha symptoms in response to years of VP symptoms (secondary).

Why do we care? Well, because truly resolving the situation involves addressing the primary imbalance that the body is mounting the secondary response to. For example, I would need to solve the dry and inflamed sinuses for my body to stop sending mucus to my sinuses. In the interim, I can also use tools to decrease the secondary sinus congestion. Similarly, I'd have to solve the dry cracked skin for my body to stop producing calloused skin, and as I do so, I can also remove the callous. With secondary imbalances, we want to address *both* the primary and the secondary imbalances.

This is a bit of an advanced topic, and not necessary for starting your personal practice of Ayurveda. I offer it here because it helps people to understand why they may have Kapha symptoms despite having few sources of Kapha coming in through life.

Balancing, Ayurveda-style

Let's get into how we approach balancing in Ayurveda. It's so wise, so simple, and so complex at the same time: We decrease the imbalance by decreasing the *dosha* that is in excess. We decrease the *doshas* by bringing in the opposite qualities. Cultivating the opposite qualities to those seen in your Current State of imbalance is how you head back to homeostasis.

Opposites balance.

For example, someone with P imbalance would soothe that state by bringing in *any* qualities opposite to those in P (e.g. cool, soft, sweet). This reduces the net P energy coming in. Bringing in the opposite qualities reduces the degree, depth, duration, and/or frequency of imbalance.

Since everything is energy, there are infinite ways to shift energy. This means I can shift the qualities of any aspect of my life in many creative ways. Say I wanted to bring in more warmth to balance V. Traditional Ayurveda may discuss warming spices, herbs, or oils. Nontraditional ways to bring in warmth, such as an herbal hot pack, aromatherapy, infrared sauna, hot yoga, being held, heating pads, and jacuzzis would also be effective ways to bring in opposite qualities to V. Once you understand the qualities you are aiming for, you can get funky with how you bring them in. The more ways you bring in desired qualities, the more quickly you decrease your imbalance.

Looking at this from our big-picture perspective, the chart below summarizes balancing approaches for VPK.

Chart 6.2 Big-picture balancing approaches for each *dosha*

Dosha	Imbalances show up as	Balancing approaches
V	degeneration, depletion, irregularity	rejuvenation, cultivating regularity, decreasing exposure to what's depleting
P	inflammation, infection	anti-inflammation
K	accumulation, stagnation, blockage	clearing, cleansing, stimulating

Balancing multiple imbalances

Let's say I have two *doshas* out of balance, like Vata and Kapha. Then I look for the qualities that are opposite to *both* Vata and Kapha (e.g. warm), and focus on bringing in those qualities in as many ways as possible. Similarly, if all three *doshas* are out of balance, I'm going to go for middle-ground choices. That's not the easiest to conceptualize, so here's an example of a middle-ground, or tridoshic balancing approach to diet:

- To balance Vata, eating food that is warm, moist and cooked— opposite to the cold, dry, and raw qualities of V in food.

- To balance Pitta, avoiding spicy hot, acidic, or fried food— decreasing the heating qualities of P.

- To balance Kapha, making sure food is not too heavy or portion sizes too big. Not heavy and not too thick to digest means food low in dairy and gluten and meat. Light and easy to digest are opposite qualities of K in food.

Pretty much anything vegetarian for lunch or dinner from any culture could fit this middle-ground set of qualities: warm, moist, cooked, not too heating, and not too much. Just like this, I look for how I can modify the qualities I'm taking in to best suit what my balancing needs are.

Additionally, we'll tailor balancing to the sources in life *through which they are coming in*. This could look like going for more V balancing in my routine if this where I have a ton of V coming in, while really focusing on reducing P in my diet if my digestion is where most of my P imbalance is. In the example of the man with multiple imbalances on page 74, we saw that bringing in opposite qualities to K would really only help in the area of food, since this was the only place it was coming in excessively.

How to approach balancing

The complexity of considering your Current State imbalances, the sources of imbalance in your life, and your Constitutional tendencies, is why we have practitioners. Even though it seems simple to bring in opposites to balance excess *dosha*, this can get easily overwhelming. Furthermore, implementation is not a thing you do—it's a lifestyle. However, a good way to begin implementing balancing is to follow the phases outlined below.

- Phase 1. Tailor daily practices.

- Phase 2. Bring in remedial measures and support.

- Phase 3. Address psychospiritual roots.

It's normal to feel overwhelmed and confused when trying to tease out how to make balancing choices. We're not used to thinking this way, and it's not a simple formula we can plug into. It really is an art of feeling and listening. Ayurveda advocates trying things out and listening to whether the symptoms get better or worse—in other words, a bit of trial and error to learn what works for you.

While we have this broad ability to shift the feeling of any energetic input, there are powerful classic ways to make sustainable shifts in Ayurveda. Namely, daily self-care practices, and remedies. In my experience, these two main categories of balancing are still the most effective. For me, all the other Ayurveda lifestyle balancing hacks are icing on the cake.

Phase 1: Balancing with daily practices

When I first came to Ayurveda, I didn't have any "daily practices." It sounded like something for monks, or old people. Now, I can't imagine life without my daily practices, and realize how important it is to start as soon in life as possible. My kids don't yet have the discipline, or interest, to do a set daily regimen, but they take herbs, saline their sinuses, and oil their bodies, as a normal part of what we do each day. They don't see it as self-care, as it's just how they were taught to do things since the beginning. I'm trying to instill in them the value of caring for your body, and emotions, every day. Not only does it have the obvious mental and physical benefits, but our inner psyche heals as we show up to value ourselves. You'll fall off your daily practices at times—that's normal, especially with travel, transition, or depletion (all V, basically). However, once you build in habits that feel good, you crave coming back to them. They help you come back into yourself, and buffer all the wear and tear of life.

Your daily self-care is not a list of things you have to do because of some Ayurveda edict. I see lots of recommendations on what to do for daily self-care, and it feels like a part time job. To me, a self-care practice is whatever combination of gestures that support your body, mind, and spirit to feel well. For this reason, I encourage you to explore all kinds of self-care practices and see what feels the best to you. This may change at times, and it's great to honor that too. On some days, a guided meditation may be part of my self-care; on others, it may be a skateboard ride by the ocean. Both leave me feeling full and inspired and connected with myself (all opposite to V), and it's nice to have some variety and flexibility to choose what feels best that day.

I'll walk you through the benefits of a daily self-care regimen in the next chapter. For now, let's consider the regimen as a primary focus for balancing shifts.

Restore health inputs first.

Just as with an ailing plant we're going to make sure it has the basics in place to thrive—sunlight, soil, water—before getting into micronutrients. If we give the plant fancy fertilizers and it doesn't have water, sun, and soil, it's unlikely to heal. For this reason, we restore the basics for health first—routine, food, self-care. And we do this before bringing in the fancy herbs and treatments. It's amazing to see how much the body heals itself when well supported with what it needs to thrive.

If you are in a place where you don't have any major symptoms, and you just have some trends that you're noticing in your Current State, then you can likely just make shifts to your daily self-care regimen. Shifting your daily routines, food, and self-care practices can be enough to significantly shift how you feel. In Ayurveda, we understand that your daily practices are the foundational inputs to your health and life. With solid daily practices and rhythms, we can balance most mild, and not yet chronic, symptoms. So this is where we start.

Our routine, food intake, and self-care practices are the major components of our daily energetic intake. Within each of these categories, there are several targets for balancing shifts. I've listed a few examples below.

- *Routine:* wake and sleep rhythms, work and rest rhythms, transitions, commuting, time with yourself

- *Food:* reduce imbalanced *doshas*, increase balancing qualities, how you eat, eating rhythms, support digestive capacity, decrease build up in the digestive tract

- *Self-care:* neti, nasya, oiling, yoga, breathwork, meditation, journaling, oracle cards, exercise.

I can brainstorm how to shift the qualities in any of the targets above to balance any *dosha*, or combination of *doshas*.

Phase 2: Balancing with remedial measures

After establishing daily practices that are supportive for health, we can bring in remedial practices. When layered on top of a supportive lifestyle, these remedial measures can be really potent. When you do any of these without the supportive daily practices, they have less impact, and less sustainable results. The three major categories of remedial practices are herbs, body therapeutics, and emotional therapeutics.

Herbs are gentle in comparison to pharmaceuticals. But they can be combined artfully to restore health while reducing symptoms in any part of the body. Most herbs also have benefits for the mind and subtle energetic body. We use herbs to balance the depletion, inflammation, or accumulation with VPK imbalances. I'll take a moment here to make a few important points about herbal supplements.

Rejuvenation is always a part of the therapeutic goals

In Ayurveda, our goal with herbs is always to support the tissues to allow them to return to full health, not simply to supplement. For example, we would rather replenish the digestive system so it can produce sufficient digestive enzymes, than simply supplement with digestive enzymes. Of course, as we are replenishing, we can enhance digestive power because we know there aren't enough digestive enzymes, but that's a short-term goal. We'd rather have the digestive system happy and healthy and doing what it does naturally best. In this case, an ideal herbal blend would be one that increases digestive power, and rejuvenates the digestive system at the same time. Every one of my formulations includes rejuvenation for the systems I'm addressing.

Multi-herb approaches are safer and more effective

We use formulas that approach the situation from multiple angles, work synergistically, and prevent side effects. If I just use neem, for example, to cool Pitta acne in the skin, I can overshoot, resulting in too much cooling, which would show as Vata signs in my digestion, like constipation. Rather, I'll use the neem and combine it with other herbs that will support it, and prevent overshooting.

Herbs need to be fresh to be potent

Herbs are only medicinal grade within a certain time frame from harvest. Just like vegetables, they lose their life force, or *prana*, over time. Beyond this time, herbs are useful for cooking and flavoring, but are not strong enough to be medicinal.

Whole herbs work best

In Ayurveda, we honor plants as living beings, and understand that a great part of their healing effect in our food and herbal formulations is their life force, or *prana*. We also know that living beings cannot be distilled down to one thing. I am not just a doctor, or just a mother, or just a writer. And it's the combination of all of my skills and talents as a doctor, mother, and writer that likely make me an effective translator for Ayurveda. Similarly, each herb has multiple skills and talents, and we are super naive in our understanding of the synergy of all the components.

We don't know how all the other parts of turmeric synergize to make the curcumin effective. This is why we use the whole herb, in all of its glory and wisdom, instead of extracts of "active ingredients."

There are lovely Ayurvedic practices to address ailments in specific parts of the body. For example we have a ghee treatment for tired eyes and migraines; vaginal herbal douches; sinus oils, joint treatments, herbal enemas.

Yes, we oil *every* orifice. The point is, for any specific ailment, there are ways to physically bring in the opposite qualities.

The Spa industry has a lot of Ayurveda terms and herbs in their marketing, and treatments may provide a nice experience. However, these are usually not traditional Ayurvedic therapeutics, which you can find in clinical settings with practitioners.

Emotional therapeutics is the part that has been dehydrated out of modern Ayurveda, and the part I'm hoping to revive. Ayurveda offers practices for emotional healing, building awareness, and helps us tie in what we are feeling with what's happening in our bodies. We'll go into this more in Chapter 9: Emotional Wellness.

Here are a few examples of balancing targets in Ayurvedic remedies:

- *Herbs:* restore doshic balance, rejuvenate affected tissues

- *Body therapeutics:* aroma, marma treatment, basti, shirodhara, etc.

- *Emotional therapeutics:* relationship dynamics, personal growth, self acceptance, life purpose, aligned decision making, internal conflicts.

With any of these three arenas of remedies, you see results with time and consistency. Just like yoga, and this is why I consider Ayurveda a lifestyle.

Phase 3: Balancing with psychospiritual practices

In Ayurveda, pathogenesis progresses from the subtle energetic body to the physical body. The first signs of imbalance would be in the *chakras* and flow of *prana* through the nadis—aka the life force moving around us that we cannot see. Most of us don't sense anything at this level, and continue life as usual. Then, the imbalances progress into the mind and emotional system. We have unpleasant feelings. If ignored, the imbalances continue their progression into the physical tissues, starting with digestive and nervous systems.

Simply stated, if we are free of internal conflict, feel connected to a life purpose, have healthy relationships, feel loved, and are in touch with our emotional needs and meeting them, our body tissues are really supported. Without these fundamentals for psychospiritual wellbeing in place, the body is taking on all the imbalances, and we're going to see physical symptoms at some point.

For deeper and more sustainable healing effects on the physical body, we'd make sure to also address the pyschospiritual underpinnings of the issue. I'll share a personal story to give you an idea of what this could look like:

I have a herniated disc in my lumbar spine. Everyone in my family has this issue. It first came on for me after becoming a mother, and then would flare on occasion. The situation was easily explained by physical strain of labor, carrying young kids around, and genetic predisposition.

Soon, the measures I used to address my physical body (chiropractors, yoga, massage, and salt baths) only subdued it temporarily, and I was told surgery was the only option. This is when I brought in measures for my emotional body: Shamanic plant ceremony, health intuitive readings, Reiki, and started correlating my emotional states preceding the flare-ups. All this lead to the awareness of the emotional root of my issue: *feeling like I have to solve everything, alone.* Sure enough, the low back is correlated with our sense of stability and security, especially financial. The right side where mine would flare has to do with my relationship with the masculine—so both with men in my life, and being too much in my own masculine energetic, over my feminine energetic.

I learned that to support a healthy back for me, I needed to ensure I felt supported, safe, and financially stable. I learned how important it was for me to not solve, and not pressure myself to solve, and began learning the art of receiving, allowing and being more in my receptive feminine. Of course, I also used physical measures, such as working with a trainer to strengthen muscles supporting the spine, pelvis, and low back.

To this day, I haven't had the surgery, but I did operate on my life. I left my marriage in the process of doing what I needed to heal the psychospiritual roots of my issues. It still flares a bit when I go through similar experiences, but I've realigned, and the flares are not as bad and much less frequent, and last about a day or two. As soon as I shift my perspectives and emotional state, I do notice a difference in my physical symptoms.

I'm not advocating divorce, or maybe I am. Either way, that's not the point. The point is that doing the deeper work to address the psychospiritual roots of your physical ailments is possible and effective. Again, this is advanced practice. I want to provide a window into what's possible down the road.

Narrowing your balancing focus

What I will walk you through in the next few chapters is a more narrow scope, and more clear direction, on balancing in the two areas most impactful on our sense of wellbeing: emotions and digestion.

Start with your heart and your gut.

First let's simplify by focusing on symptoms in digestion and emotional body. Then, let's see if we can go for the source directly, and bring in opposite qualities in as many ways as we can imagine. Starting with the easiest changes first gets us on the path with some momentum; even if they are gentle baby steps they will create shifts over time. Every step counts.

- Focus on digestive and emotional symptoms. (We'll explore why in the next chapter.)

- Go for the source of the imbalance as directly as possible.

- Start with the easiest shifts.

I'll walk you through these considerations, and a few others, that will help you get clear on what you need in the *Balancing Check-In* (Appendix 5).

Common misperceptions about balancing

*Each **dosha** has qualities which may balance the other two*

To balance Vata, we want the opposite qualities of Vata. Oftentimes people recognize that the depleting effects of Vata are opposite to the rejuvenative effects of Kapha, and start to say "I need more Kapha to balance my Vata." In reality, there are aspects of each of the *doshas* that balance the other two. There are qualities of both P and K that

are opposite, or balancing, for V. There are qualities of both P and V
that are opposite, or balancing, for K. There are qualities of both V and
K that are opposite, or balancing for P.

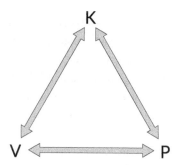

Figure 6.2 *Each* dosha *has qualities opposite to the other two* doshas

You can't do this alone

(I tried!) We all need each other. We are relational beings. We help each
other "see" the patterns in our lives and support each other through
shifting them. I can't heal myself. Not that I don't have the ability to see
energetics and shift them. But I can't see from within the energetics of my
life what someone can from the outside. I'm too entrenched.

Sustainability requires support, and mostly from yourself.

Balancing is a skill, like learning to be happy, that we have to teach
ourselves and have a lot of support for over time. We get better and better
at it, but it's not something that we can stop doing. Over time, we do
need less support because we become clearer on our patterns and more
confident in our ability to shift them.

Until then, bring in support. You're stepping into a new way of seeing
life and responding to it. That takes support. I hope you'll stay connected
with Ayurveda, and bring in any and all supports for your balancing
changes. Maybe that's working with me. Maybe that's a therapist and
a personal trainer and a nutritionist. It doesn't matter what support
you bring in, as long as you feel supported in shifting the energetics of
your life.

For remedial therapeutics, you'll want to work with an experienced
practitioner.

Change requires work

I could put together a list of practices to reduce Vata, Pitta, and Kapha, and most of us won't change our experience even with that list of remedies. Why? Well, because change requires work, and work requires energy and time. Expecting yourself to go against your long-term patterns and imbalances without having time and energy carved out is not realistic.

I think it's important to acknowledge here that this shift happens in bite-size steps. You do what you can, and I'll keep reminding you that every step counts. Let's say my aim is to cook all my food and be entirely processed-food-free. But, in my current reality, I'm eating out several times a week and reheating leftovers in the microwave at work. That's a big jump to make in lifestyle. Likely there are factors in place that are why my current reality doesn't match my desired one. However, starting with switching to glass tupperware is a valuable step. Cooking one or two times more per week is another valuable step. Choosing to eat vegetarian when I eat out is another great step. Slowly, over time, I'm taking steps towards my goal. This is how most sustainable change happens.

Similarly, few people in the Western world have a health-promoting foundation of daily practices. Restructuring your daily rhythms, food, and self-care practices *is a big deal*. It doesn't just happen overnight, and last. When it happens slowly over time, it's truly a shift in lifestyle—just like yoga.

The power of healing choices

In Vedic wisdom, we choose every experience we have, either consciously or subconsciously. Our choices affect our bodies, minds, and spirits. This is hard to digest because we don't like to see ourselves as responsible for, or having chosen, the traumatic experiences we've had. In Vedic philosophy, traumatic experiences, like the healing ones, like *all* experiences, happen for a reason—*to be catalysts of our spiritual growth*. When we apply our awareness to make conscious decisions, it has a healing effect.

All of our experiences are opportunities to gain clarity of what we truly want in life, to become wiser, to learn to operate in a way that is in alignment with what we wish to experience. When we take advantage of these opportunities, we have greater awareness. Spiritual growth is cultivating and applying this awareness.

Spiritual growth = applied awareness

Here's an example of the interconnections between increased awareness, conscious decision making (aka spiritual growth), and health:

A woman has a minor car accident. She was late and frantically looking up directions to her destination (and she hadn't put on her makeup yet, or eaten breakfast).

Instead of her usual response (getting frustrated, judging herself and building her anxiety), she chose to see the lessons and areas for growth in the experience. She gained clarity that she didn't want to endanger herself, or others, because she is rushing and stressed; that she doesn't want the experience of feeling rushed or stressed at all; that she really wants to feel more organized and prepared and in ease.

She chose to view the car accident as the vehicle (pun intended) for her to learn to really prioritize her feeling organized, prepared, and at ease over other experiences she had been prioritizing (sleeping in, staying up late watching TV, picking up a call from her mom, etc.).

In Vedic wisdom, we would say that she had learned a karmic lesson of greater self-love. By learning how to show up for her intentions with her decisions, words, and actions, she now had less internal conflict, which heals the subtle energetic body.

Her shift into really prioritizing being prepared and not rushed, feeling safe and on top of things, also resulted in less adrenal fatigue, better digestion and immunity, and greater self-worth. In this particular example, she reduced the Vata in her experience so she also reduced the frequency/intensity/presence of all Vata symptoms in her body, which happened to be poor memory, fatigue, night waking, and menstrual cramps.

It's all so interconnected. Our life affects all of who we are, the body and everything beyond the body. Our choices to heal will too. Healing happens on every level when you finally prioritize *how you feel*.

Summary

- Imbalance is a state of excess.

- Multiple imbalances can occur simultaneously.

- Imbalances begin in the subtle body, and then take root in the physical body.

- Balance too much VPK by bringing in more of the opposite qualities of VPK in any aspect of life.

- Target sources of imbalance when possible.

- Start with digestion and emotional balancing.

- Daily practices make remedial measures successful.

You can probably get a sense of your personal balancing needs already. I've put together some reflective questions in the *Balancing Check-In* (Appendix 5) to help walk you through considerations which will shed light on your path to balance. These are questions and considerations I ask myself regularly, not just once. Remember, balancing is a lifelong practice with ups and downs. You will take a few steps forward, and a few steps back, and it's all moving forward actually.

Chapter 7

START HERE

Overview of Where to Begin
Implementing in Your Life, and Why

Learning objectives

- Understand why digestion and emotions are a good starting place for balancing.

- Get a feeling for Ayurvedic lifestyle.

Even though "where am I at, what do I need?" seems like a simple self inquiry process, it's broad and ambiguous. On top of that, we're not used to feeling qualified to answer that question. For these reasons, many students have found it helpful to have a narrower, clear, and defined scope within which to begin this practice.

When I think of the most impactful place to start, the answer is clear: *emotional wellness and digestion.* In the next two chapters, I'll lay out specific tools to help observe and respond to emotional and digestive patterns in real time. Here, I'd like to build our collective awareness of why that is, and what it accomplishes for you.

Why start with emotional patterns?

In Ayurveda, and most ancient perspectives, imbalances begin in the subtle energetic body—at the level of spirit and emotions. In the many different holistic sciences and cultures, the common thread is that imbalance begins in the non-physical parts of us and then progresses into the physical parts of us.

In the West, we are in our infancy in understanding the nature of the relationship between the emotional body and the physical body. Ayurveda, Traditional Chinese Medicine, Shamanism, and other holistic healing sciences have a sophisticated understanding of the relationship between our life purpose, our internal conflicts, our emotions, and our physical experience. What we have clearly proven with modern research is that emotions affect the body. Good feeling emotions support healing in the physical body. Unpleasant emotional states promote disease progression and degeneration. In other words, we cannot really be healthy without feeling good emotionally—it's a prerequisite, or an integral component, of feeling well.

We cannot really be healthy if we're not happy.

Since the inception of imbalance occurs in the non-physical, there is not a complete healing until the psychospiritual roots have been attended to in any physical ailment. Oftentimes the emotional patterns are lifelong and from our childhood imprint—they aren't always going to be quick to shift. In fact, it's likely to take years to shift emotional patterns of how you receive and respond to your life experience. However, even hanging that "in progress" sign on your emotional imbalances does help to create a lot of peace and empowerment, and ultimately, health. The idea is that we are working to start healing in the body, decrease symptoms, all while starting to address the root causes.

In the first chapter, I spoke of modern presentations of Ayurveda as "dehydrated" of emotional wellness. Not including emotional wellness renders Ayurveda less effective. I've heard many stories where people recount their disappointment with the effects of an herbal supplement or week-long cleanse. Bluntly stated, if you have a lot of ongoing stress and internal conflict, there is no herb or superfood or cleanse that is going to be able to protect your body from the effects of that. Now, when we go for a comprehensive solution, such as one that includes emotional healing, self-care practices, diet and herbal support for the body, and awareness building to make healthier choices, the healing shifts are guaranteed.

In summary, the benefits of beginning your Ayurvedic practice with emotional pattern awareness are:

- addressing the root causes of physical ailments
- creating fertile ground for health in the physical body

- increasing the effectiveness of remedial balancing measures (e.g. herbs, diet).

Why start with digestive patterns?

I view the digestive system as one of the main portals through which the energetics of the emotional body come into the physical body. All parts of our bodies are affected by our emotions, and we can feel the effects of stress in many ways, from muscle tension to irritability to decreased immunity. However, the first place we see the effects of the emotional body on the physical systems is in the digestive system. It makes sense, then, that digestion presents the first signs of excessive, or imbalanced, *doshas* in the body. By balancing our digestive patterns, we can catch energetic shifts in our physical body *before* they progress into deeper tissues.

The digestive system is, ultimately, a massive processing and distribution center for the body. Everything in the digestive system, not only nutrients, but also excess *dosha* and toxic build-up, gets poured into the bloodstream, and thus, delivered to *all* parts of the body. So, healthy digestion ensures that what is getting sent to the body tissues is optimal nutrition, and as little imbalance as possible. Optimizing digestion is the most potent preventive medicine, as the entire body is so dependent on digestive health. This is why Ayurveda places so much emphasis on healthy digestion.

All disease begins in the gut. (Hippocrates)

Research now shows that most of the diseases of modern living begin in the gut and are related to our diet. The gut-brain is a superhighway with many lanes of information traffic going in either direction between the brain in the head and the brain in the belly. Mental and emotional stress triggers physical responses that affect the gut, while disturbances in the microbiome—the colony of microorganisms in the gut—affect the functioning and the health of the brain. When the gut colony becomes unbalanced with more harmful microorganisms than helpful ones, the flora in the belly begin to produce toxins that wreak havoc with the immune system, alter brain function and mood, and weaken immune defenses.[1]

---

1   Villoldo (2015, p.36)

Even in modern medicine, most all chronic digestive ailments are correlated with emotional states. Even though the gut-brain connection is a hot area of research in the West, we still don't have clear answers as to *how* emotions relate to specific pathology. In Ayurveda, we do. The emotions correlated with digestive ailments are related in their qualities, and *doshas*. In other words, P emotions are found with P digestive imbalances; V digestive issues always come with V emotions and mind-states; K digestive symptoms are seen with signs of K in the mind and emotions. Because we stay distracted, over-stimulated, and prioritize other things, we often are unaware of our emotional state. As you become aware of digestive patterns which are easier to witness, you'll naturally increase your awareness of emotional states.

Our Current State digestive patterns result from our Constitutional tendencies interacting with current life energetics. Everyone knows their own personal response to stress in their digestive features. Some of us get constipated with stress, while others need to keep running to the toilet; some eat more when they are nervous, while nervousness in others shows as decreased appetite. As you witness your patterns, you'll now be able to start to understand them in the context of VPK.

Once you get into observing your patterns, and exploring the causes, you'll start to see the correlation of the emotions, of the foods, and of the energetic environs in which you eat. If I was to put numbers to what I'm seeing with clients, I'd say about 50 percent of digestive symptomatology is due to unpleasant feelings (stress); perhaps 30 percent due to the energetics of the food; and about 20 percent due to the energetics of how we eat. Our emotional state largely governs our true digestive capacity— what your digestion can handle when happy and healthy is different to when you are when upset or depleted.

This is quite different from the Western viewpoint that all that is happening in the digestive system is mainly due to what we eat. I know plenty of people that are gluten free, dairy free, meat free, etc. and still experience digestive symptoms. Their symptoms may have improved greatly with diet change, however, they still often present with digestive patterns that reveal imbalance. Simply avoiding triggering foods is not a complete remedy. There is so much to be said about digestion from the Ayurvedic lens, and there are many good books and cookbooks dedicated to this topic. For our purposes, a focus on digestive wellness serves us in many ways:

- It reveals the first signs of changes in energetics.

- It relates to, and further reveals, emotional states.

- It provides feedback on what we are eating and how we are eating.

- Healthy digestion supports every other tissue system.

Your life affects your emotions, which in turn greatly affects your digestive health, which in turn affects the rest of you. In the short term, we'll step into the greater vision of Ayurvedic lifestyle by taking a few strides towards digestive and emotional health. Perhaps more importantly, we're heading towards greater self awareness, and recognizing some of our patterns across life, emotions, and digestion. Over time, these patterns will become familiar dialogue between you and your body, and you'll converse with them in ease.

Reverent connected lifestyle

I think of the women in ancient Indus Valley matriarchal agricultural societies doing *chandra sadhana*, bleeding on the fields to tailor the nutrient profile of their crops; informing their pineal glands by placing their menses on their *bindu* (third eye point) and thus modulating their reproductive tissues and their *shakti* (manifestational potency). This is so beyond taking ashwagandha supplements and doing a Vinyasa level ⅔ class a few times a week.

This is reverent, connected. Everything in Ayurveda is about honoring the connections: our minds with our hearts, our emotional bodies with our physical bodies; ourselves and others; ourselves and nature. In fact, aligning our lifestyle with the rhythms of the natural universe has a healing effect on the body. Facets of Ayurvedic daily rhythms and self-care are called *dinacharya*, and form the backbone of Ayurvedic lifestyle. I don't want to give you a blueprint on how to live your day, like rules to follow. That would be contrary to our approach. Instead, I'll mention the natural rhythms to align with in our balancing practices in digestion and emotions.

We're missing the spiritual growth, community, ritual, accountability, wise elders, and all the parts of the human experience that promote emotional integration. So we seek it in self-help books, TED talks, therapists, and yoga teachers. The breakdown of community structure in modern urban life highlights the importance of being connected to our inner guidance, nature, and others on this path. If you are plugged into yourself, and your emotional and digestive patterns, you'll feel the benefits of this greater state of connection to yourself. You'll start choosing differently, more healthfully, simply because you're paying more attention.

The figure below outlines my view of Ayurvedic lifestyle. We're regularly checking in with ourselves and the qualities we are feeling. If those qualities are feeling good, we are validated that our choices are energetically beneficial for us. If there are qualities that do not feel good, that's our simple signal light to choose our energetics differently. It's a conscious lifestyle because it requires operating in deeper awareness and choosing the best energetics for ourselves and our personal environs.

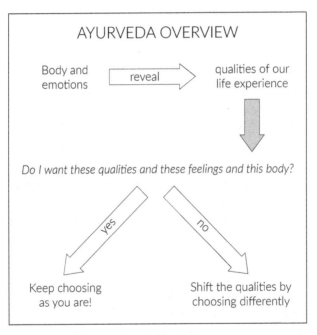

Figure 7.1 *Ayurvedic decision making*

The power of one shift

In the next two chapters, I'll present ways to interpret patterns in these two systems, and several tools. You may be motivated to try to overhaul your patterns and implement as many shifts as possible. I did that. Then I overwhelmed myself, and went back to default patterns.

I decided, instead, to go deeper into an experience by narrowing my breadth—in other words, the whole quality over quantity approach. The more energy we have going in different directions, the more energy is dispersed amongst those many directions. When you decrease the number of directions you're shooting energy out to, the intensity of the remaining rays increases—you have a more full experience. This is why I'd love for you to experience what simply one shift feels like. Of course, when applied consistently. I'd recommend applying any shift for at least two weeks. As all the suggestions in this book are gentle and natural they need time to show effects.

The first shift I'd suggest is to create the space for this practice. We need time to be able to check in with ourselves and think, and feel, out our choices. Ideally, you'd have at least an hour to yourself each day. As you know from yoga, it feels so good to have time alone to get out of your brain and into your body; to release mental and physical tension; to be in gratitude. Ideally, we'd do a self check in from this present, sacred space. That takes me about one-and-a-half hours a day. It's not particularly easy to have this much time in modern life, I know. But I feel the difference when I don't give this to myself, and it never feels good. When I have a languid two hours to check in with myself, I'm glowing. I'd say 30 minutes a day is the bare minimum for sanity. If you don't already have daily "me" time, you'll have to create that. It's the altar upon which we can practice Ayurveda.

Your "daily 30"

One of the most foundational steps you can take towards Ayurvedic lifestyle is creating some time and space every day to be with yourself.

Do something to get out of your head. Whatever works for you is fine. So-hum chanting, *Pranayama*, stretching, listening to a guided meditation. Anything that allows you to not be in an active state for anything other than self dialogue.

Then simply ask yourself how you are feeling. Write down some qualities. Try to identify *doshas* present in the qualities you are feeling. Ask yourself what you need to feel good that day.

Morning is best, as it's the Kapha time of day, and a fertile time for spiritual practices. However, anytime is fine! See if you can commit to a solid "daily 30" as a lifestyle in which you have as much time to check in with yourself as you spend on countless less important things.

Summary

This is not a cookbook, a guide to enlightenment, or a comprehensive review of digestive assessment and treatment. It's a starting place for a personal journey to support your digestion of your food, and your emotional experience. In summary, we're going for emotional and digestive wellness because:

- these systems affect all other systems in the body, in a big way

- emotional and digestive signs and patterns are easy to observe

- they show changes in real time. As emotional and digestive patterns are the fastest to respond to life energetics, they give us the most rapid signs of shifts in energy

- for the same reason, these are also the easiest systems to implement tools for.

Chapter 8

DIGESTIVE WELLNESS

Learning objectives

- Understand the concept of digestive capacity.

- Learn about what makes foods more digestible.

- Begin to sense what your digestive system is communicating.

- Get a sense of how to match the energetics of your food to your digestive needs.

- Learn healthy eating habits which benefit regardless of your Current State.

In the West, we put so much emphasis on *what* we are eating as the cause of our digestive state. While it's true that what you are eating affects your digestive system, as I mentioned in the last chapter, that's only part of the picture.

There is information to support, and negate, every approach to food. Frankly, the information and focus on what to eat is overwhelming and confusing. *Is kombucha good, or bad? Which probiotics are best? What about "gut shots" and are carbohydrates really okay to eat? Should we be vegan and entirely plant-based? Is bone broth just as effective in a protein powder?* The considerations are never-ending, as are the expert opinions on all of these topics. Just knowing what to eat could be a part time research job that leads to inconclusive results.

The reason we cannot find any one sure way to eat that is "right" or "best" is because different people need different things. A tall, muscular, athletic man with a very high metabolism and activity level has different needs than a sedentary, short man with more fat than muscle. A teenage girl has different needs than a menopausal woman. Someone with a Pitta predominance in their Constitution has different needs than someone with a Kapha predominance.

Furthermore, what we need from our food is always changing. The qualities that would be balancing for me in food are different in the morning, midday, and evening; during times of high stress or ease; during the summer versus winter; during menses and ovulation.

What we are missing, in a huge way, is the ability to know *what our bodies are wanting from our food*. And this is where I would like to focus. Ayurveda's wisdom on digestion could fill volumes. My goal is to give you the ability to begin to sense what your digestive system is communicating to you, so you can better feel what it needs at that moment.

Digestive capacity

One of the most important ways to "hear" our digestive system is to be aware of digestive capacity, or *agni*. *Agni* is often translated as "fire" and fire is regarded as a transformative force. As we discussed with our exploration of Pitta *dosha*, fire takes whatever it is burning and transforms it into heat and light energy. Every tissue system in the body has a transformative function, where it takes some substrate and turns it into the product of that system—bone, blood, neural connections, memories, vaginal secretions, enzymes, etc. With the digestive system, *agni* is the transformative force that takes your food and transforms it into the micronutrients that your body needs. You may have heard the term "*agni*" in your yoga training, as there are several postures and practices to improve it. In digestion, regard *agni* as your digestive capacity. Think of it as your metabolism, appetite, and digestive enzymes rolled into one concept.

Ideally, we want to match our food intake with our capacity to digest. That makes sense. The problem is that our brains and habits get in the way—we don't eat when we're hungry because we're too busy, or we eat mindlessly in front of the computer. We don't eat enough. We eat too much. We choose foods based on the amount of carbs, or perceived health benefit, or cravings, instead of on the ability of our body to digest it. One of my students summed up our collective experience brilliantly, "I don't know what to do about food. Who does? I mean, having your food figured out is like witchcraft." She's right. It's not simple, and it's a moving target.

However, there are some basic approaches to digestive wellness that have helped me a great deal in how I operate with food and eating. I'll share these basics and the reasons why they are effective, and you can choose to incorporate what you are drawn to.

Listening to your appetite

We cannot really sense our metabolism or digestive enzyme levels, but we can sense appetite. This is why it's the best proxy for sensing your digestive capacity, or *agni*. Developing a close relationship with your appetite is a great way to know when, what, and how much to eat. Simply stated, eat when you are physically hungry, and don't eat when you are not. Eat heavier foods and larger portions when you have a strong appetite; eat lighter foods and smaller portions when you don't. Don't let the basic nature of this wisdom let you think it's not powerful, or easy to implement.

When we have a healthy digestive capacity, and eat food that it can handle well, the food is completely digested. It's akin to a good fire burning cleanly through the wood placed in it. If you put too many logs, or too dense wood, on a weak fire, it may go out and leave behind partially burned wood. Similarly, when we eat more than our digestive capacity, there is partially digested food left over. This partially digested food then ferments and becomes toxic build-up in our digestive tract. We call this build-up *ama* in Ayurveda and nitrogenous waste in Western medicine. If you have build-up, it will be distributed to the rest of the body, alongside everything else the digestive system is delivering to tissues. Eventually, *ama* lodges itself and accumulates in your vulnerable tissues—the joints, the nerves, the thyroid, etc. As *ama* accumulates in any part of the body, the immune system begins to attack it, and there is inflammation. This is the basis of all auto-immune phenomena according to Ayurveda, and it's a serious and common process underlying so many diseases. Over burdening our digestive systems doesn't lead to anything good, and overconsumption is largely responsible for the rise in all diseases associated with urbanization.

Your digestive capacity is directly influenced by your Current State imbalances and your emotional state. When you are working intensely and building up a lot of Pitta in the mind, and feeling intense, your appetite increases. When you are traveling, or fighting a cold, it decreases. We're talking about your true physical "my-stomach-is-growling" appetite here, not an emotional or mental one.

In general:

- When there are mostly Pitta imbalances in the body and mind, you'll experience a hyper-strong appetite and metabolism. Food is really important and you don't skip meals. You get irritable, "hangry," if you have to wait to eat, and can dip into hypoglycemic states. You may have snacks on deck because of this, and need to eat a bit of something every two to three hours.

- When there are mostly Kapha imbalances in the body and mind, you'll experience less appetite, and slow digestion. In the morning especially, there is low appetite, and one big meal a day feels sufficient with some snacks and drinks. There may be a tendency towards late night snacking and sweet cravings.

- When there are mostly Vata imbalances in the body and mind, you'll experience low, or extreme fluctuations of appetite. It could be like you didn't even think of food for half a day, and then suddenly, you're famished. However, you get full fast, and distracted from food easily.

Of course, these are generalizations, and you can have combinations of features when you have more than one *dosha* imbalance. When you don't "fit in a box" description is when things start to feel tricky and unclear. For this reason, I think it's more effective to just check in with your tummy.

Before you eat, ask yourself if you have a true appetite

We all eat emotionally. We're hardwired this way as humans. Babies nurse not only when they are hungry, but also when they are tired, uncomfortable, or stressed. Dairy, sugar, and chocolate all help to release the same anandamides in the brain that nursing does when we are babies, which is why ice cream and desserts are commonly what we reach for to self-soothe. But cravings can run the spectrum from salty or crunchy to foods we have assigned in our memories as comfort foods. The key here is to know when you are eating to fuel, or eating to soothe. If you are eating to fuel the vehicle of your body, proceed to the next consideration. When eating to soothe, focus on something light and easy to digest. Maybe that's a warm nut milk with some spices (vanilla, cardamom, cinnamon), or soup, or fruit, or a scrambled egg. What it is doesn't matter, as much as keeping it easy to digest. Just be present, and allow yourself to feel as soothed as possible. This prevents mindless overeating and burdening our digestive systems.

Ask yourself what qualities would feel good to consume

Heavy, light, moist, dry, salty, sweet, alkaline, tart, etc.? I like to close my eyes, put my right hand on my belly, and ask it what it really feels like consuming. This is just a simple practice for me to get away from my brain choosing my food. Another trick I use is to imagine how I would feel while eating what I'm about to choose, and after eating it. Most often, my belly will give me a yes, or no, about the choice I'm imagining.

Is my body really hungry?

What feels balancing to my body right now?

With the above two check-ins, we are connecting to our true appetite, the root of our "hunger," and understanding what our bodies are really wanting to feel good. This is all towards greater self awareness, and will naturally, organically, lead to food choices that are better matched to your digestive capacity.

This is surprisingly scary and difficult for many people. They don't trust what they feel, and just want rules and meal plans. All that is easily found online. What I'll encourage is that you try these practices out, even if you are choosing your food based on some strategy. We can always practice feeling more, even when not quite ready to act on the awareness of those feelings.

Connecting to the energetics of your food

As we've been discussing throughout this book, food is a big energetic input. In Chapter 3, we looked at the basic qualities of your food in the *VPK in My Life Worksheet* (Appendix 1). Here we were just practicing identifying qualities and the *doshas* those qualities reveal in this major arena of your life. We can do this same practice every time we put something in our mouths. Literally, you can sense the qualities of anything you are eating, and figure out the *doshas* you are taking in. If I'm having a sandwich, and it feels dry in my mouth, there must be Vata coming in from that sandwich. If it also feels dense, or heavy, in my stomach, then there must also be Kapha coming in with that sandwich. The qualities you feel more are the ones more present.

As we discussed in balancing approaches, we choose opposite qualities to balance. So, if you have a lot of Vata imbalances, you want to eat less food that has Vata qualities, and more food that has opposite to Vata qualities. Let's say I wake up one morning feeling heavy-headed and sluggish (K). On that day I may want to incorporate a more K balancing approach to food. Let's say the next day I'm feeling depleted and with Vata signs of imbalance in my digestion and muscles and emotions. Then, I'd shift into a more Vata balancing approach.

Once you get good at sensing your Current State in the morning, and approaching your food accordingly that day, you can start to get even more detailed. I could start the day feeling congested and with low appetite (K), and then shift into more intensity, irritability, with a strong appetite (P) around midday; and feel gassy, bloated, and restless (V) in the evening. In this case, I'd start with a K balancing approach in the morning, shift into a more P balancing approach midday, and end with a V balancing approach for the evening.

Digestibility

Charts are helpful for quick reference, and reminding ourselves about healing approaches. I also want to provide the "why" behind these suggestions so that you are increasing your knowledge and awareness. In general, all food is easier to digest when it's warm, moist, cooked, and seasoned. Cooking and seasoning helps to predigest food. The digestive tract actually spasms and "turns off" with cold foods and drinks. The stomach works best on foods that match its environs—warm in temperature and moist.

Foods that are clean (no weird chemicals or preservatives) are easier to digest. Foods that are heaviest to digest are dense and feel heavy in the tummy (oatmeal, mashed potatoes, beef, nut butters). There are foods with heavy or thick quality that are easy to digest such as coconut oil and ghee, and you can know this because they don't feel heavy in your belly after consumption. Lighter foods don't feel so thick in your mouth, and digest more quickly.

All culinary spices from every culture are herbs with medicinal properties that support digestion—from salt to garlic to basil to turmeric. Thus, using any culinary seasoning or spices helps to make food easier to digest. Many spices are warming in nature, and thus support *agni*. There are some that are cooling in nature that still aid digestion, such as dill, coriander, fennel, and mint.

> *Warm, moist, organic, unprocessed, seasoned, plant-based, and made with love = easy to digest*

Try to be aware of how easy to digest your food is given the above. Things that you may have viewed as healthy, such as dry protein bars, or salad, may actually be hard to digest given the above physiologics of *agni* and what the stomach likes. Dipping raw broccoli in ranch is doubly challenging for digestion, as it's cold, dry, raw, and then with heavy dairy. Apples and almond butter would be another challenging combo—raw, cold with heavy, and hard to digest. We may need to rewire our thoughts, redefining "healthy" food to include good digestibility. I've incorporated these physiologic basics in the *dosha* specific balancing approaches below.

Balancing approaches

In Chart 8.1, I summarize qualities that are balancing for Vata, Pitta, and Kapha imbalances. Additionally, I've listed out some approaches to food rhythms that attend to the classic patterns of *agni* with imbalance in each *dosha*. You can use this as a starting guide on how to approach food based on your Current State.

Chart 8.1 Signs of imbalanced *agni* and balancing approaches by *dosha*

Dosha	V	P	K
Signs of imbalanced *agni*	Forget to eat Graze all day Mindless snacking Extreme hunger after long periods of not thinking of food Get anxious or lightheaded when don't eat	Always hungry Need to eat every few hours Get angry and irritable if don't eat	Low morning appetite Don't need the classic three meals Feel okay if don't eat for long periods Feel heavy and sleepy after eating Sluggish digestion

cont.

Balancing approaches			
Qualities of food to increase	Warm Moist Cooked Seasoned Grounding Nourishing Fermented (in moderation)	Green / Alkaline Cooling Substantive Nutritive Slimy	Green/ Bitter Light/ easy to digest Warm Dry/ astringent (in moderation) Spicy-hot Cooked
Examples	Root vegetables Superfoods Supergrains Light, easy to digest protein All spices	Sweet fruit Greens Protein heavy grains Complex carbs Animal protein Cooling spices	Warming spices Cooked veggies Easy to digest proteins Light grains
Qualities of food to decrease	Raw Dry/ crunchy Bland Cold Dairy Heavy	Spicy-hot Fermented Acidic Fried Salty Nightshades*	Heavy carbs and meat Sweet Dense Dairy
Food rhythms	Regular eating—schedule for at least three meals Greatest meal at lunch Smaller portions more frequently best	Regular meals and snacks in between Greatest meal at lunch Good solid breakfast in the morning A solid dinner	Maybe skip breakfast, or eat lightly when hunger sets in Greatest meal at lunch Lighter dinner Stop eating earlier in the evening

With Vata imbalance, we have a weakened digestive capacity due to depletion. So we want to keep everything easy to digest. This is why warm, moist, cooked, seasoned foods are best. Because digestive capacity is not really strong, avoiding really heavy and hard to digest foods is helpful in avoiding build-up of *ama*. Some of the heaviest foods are gluten, dairy

---

*   A family of vegetables including white potatoes, eggplant, tomatoes, and peppers.

(especially the modern dairy industry which is not fresh raw milk that Ayurveda advises), and meat (especially red meats). This is why a lot of people with weak *agni* end up with an acquired sensitivity to these heavier foods. I've seen many clients that identified as gluten intolerant become tolerant after increasing their digestive capacity and changing the qualities of their food intake to balance Vata. Vata imbalanced digestive capacity is also challenged by hard-to-digest foods such as lentils, nuts, and raw vegetables. These foods typically have a lot of Vata, and require pre-digestion with adequate cooking, soaking, and spicing to be friendly to a Vata state of *agni*. In summary, with Vata symptoms in digestion, you want to regard your *agni* as depleted, and make everything really easy to digest. Smaller portions work well, and eating more frequently helps to prevent against further depletion. The greatest challenge here is that almost anything you can "grab-n-eat," aka snacks, are all Vata in nature. So, having real cooked food available, and maybe eating it in multiple settings is the way to go, but that takes forethought and planning that people with Vata imbalance find challenging. Simply starting by leaning towards the qualities of warm, moist, cooked, and spiced more often is a good plan.

In terms of what to eat for Vata balancing, foods that inherently are grounding, warming, and highly nutritious are the way to go. Root vegetables and grains are good examples. Anything that you eat which you feel deeply nourished by is likely Vata reducing.

With Pitta imbalance, there is usually a strong and steady appetite. The challenge here is having to constantly feed yourself something substantial. Utilizing a more protein heavy diet and incorporating greater density (yes, carbs, dairy, and meat) helps to keep the hunger at bay. Alternatively, planning for eating every few hours with carbohydrate-based snacks, like fruit, smoothies, and oatmeal could work as well. If Pitta *agni* is not fed for several hours, the mental hunger built up over that time commonly leads to overeating. This taxes the thyroid, as the body is being forced to function without enough fuel, and then overfueled. The thyroid is the determinant of our basal metabolic rate—the rate at which we utilize our fuel. So not eating when you are hungry forces it to change to a lower metabolic rate; this followed by overeating causes a mismatch between the amount of fuel and the rate at which the body can burn it. The thyroid then has to try to increase the rate, but if you're at the end of your day and decompressing in front of the TV, it's like overfueling a parked car. Thyroid function and metabolism are complex dynamic aspects of the body. For our purposes, we need to understand that when you're hungry and don't eat, or when you overeat as a result of being hungry for a long time, it strains these systems.

I don't recommend too much cold or raw food for Pitta *agni* because these are not supportive of digestive function in general. However, if you're going to do cold or raw foods, only a Pitta strong digestive capacity can handle these occasionally, and more so when there is a lot of Pitta. So, if I'm going to eat ice cream, it's more easily handled on a hot day than in the middle of winter or in the cool of the evening. If I'm going to have salad which has raw greens in it, I can make it easier to digest by ensuring the greens are covered in oil (think massaged kale) and digestive spices. This is the wisdom behind salad dressing—oil, vinegar, salt and herbs all help to predigest the greens. So, some raw is fine for Pitta *agni*, but we can still modify to support easeful digestion.

When selecting foods for Pitta balancing, it's really about greens and alkalinity. Everything from the brassica vegetable family is wonderful for everyone, but especially those with a lot of Pitta. In addition, we want to avoid bringing in more Pitta with salty, fried, acidic (citrus), spicy-hot, or fermented foods. Yes, fermented. While sauerkraut, kimchi, apple cider vinegar, and kombucha are all being well acclaimed for their digestive benefits, they are all heating. Their heating nature is why they support *agni* and improve digestive capacity. This is great in moderation and before meals. Bringing in too much of anything fermented will increase Pitta and candida overgrowth (PK), and for this reason Vata *agni* is the one that is best prescribed fermented digestive support. High protein grains, complex carbohydrates, poultry/fish (of course optional), and legumes, are additional staples for a Pitta balancing approach because they are substantive. Sweet fruit helps to cool.

With Kapha digestive capacity, it's most important to wait to eat until you really have an appetite. Because of the dim *agni* with Kapha imbalance, we're more likely to accumulate in general, and accumulate toxic build-up in the digestive tract. For most, this means just having some form of warm liquid in the morning, and waiting a few hours until lunchtime to have a more substantive meal. As digestion is more sluggish, it takes longer to digest and there may not be a need for another big meal. Usually a lighter meal, like cooked vegetables, easy-to-digest protein, or soups will be sufficient for the evening, and are also the staples of a Kapha balancing food approach. Another challenge is to avoid the cravings for sweets, dairy, and carbs, as these tend to increase the Kapha imbalance. At the very least, go for small amounts of natural sweets which are not processed and easy to digest. Choosing an almond milk chia seed pudding, for example, would be a much better fit than commercial ice cream. There's always a way to meet your craving in a way that is less imbalancing.

Balancing digestions is like riding a unicorn.

Common misperceptions
Food charts will tell you what to eat

Food charts are fantastic for understanding the basic qualities or *doshas* in individual foods. For example, cabbage is very crunchy, and mostly hard to digest because of how much indigestible fiber it has. You may be able to sense crunch and fiber by just taking a bite of cabbage. As your sensing skills mature, you may also be able to sense the astringent, bitter, and slightly sweet nature of the cabbage. Either way, the major qualities convey Vata energy, and you'll see cabbage listed as a "Vata food," meaning you should *not* eat more of it if you have Vata imbalance. The big mistake here is to not consider how the cabbage has been modified before it enters your body. My mom's cabbage is first sauteed in ghee, cumin seeds, and fresh ginger, and then steamed until it's soft enough to melt in your mouth. It's also served warm, and has a broth to it. Thus, the qualities of the cabbage have been modified to warm, moist, cooked, and spiced and when eating her cabbage dish, I'm actually balancing Vata. Of course if a food has a lot of an energy, we'll likely sense that in the dish, such as the Kapha energy in potatoes. However, it's more important to note the qualities of the whole dish, as it enters your mouth. Most things we eat have more than one ingredient, and that means they are a mix of qualities and energies. So we need to sense the specifics of the complete dish, not the individual ingredients.

Similarly, no food chart can summarize every version of that food. Take tomatoes, for example, they are usually acidic and tart, and thus will be charted as a "Pitta food." However, my neighbor's heirlooms are sweet and watery, and don't have a hint of tartness. They clearly are less Pitta imbalancing than the average tomato. A banana will be charted as a "Kapha food" because bananas are sweet and slimy. However, an unripe banana could be very bitter and astringent (dries your mouth), which reveals Vata energy. Hopefully these examples underscore that the only way to really know what qualities and *doshas* you are eating, is to feel them in your mouth and your tummy.

Only eat certain healthy foods

When we look at food charts, or engage in specific diets, or meal plans, there is a tendency to limit our food lexicon to certain foods we've categorized in our minds as healthy, or safe, or good. Ayurveda advocates for rotating your diet, and especially eating seasonally. You may not even be in touch with what grows in what season, as supermarkets make it seem like everything is always available. Nature offers us innate balancing, as the foods that grow each season naturally have qualities that balance the energetics of that season. Citrus helps to balance the Kapha of Spring; sweet melons balance the Pitta heat of Summer; and the root vegetables of Fall counter the high Vata of Autumn and Winter. The Farmer's Market is a great way to stay in touch with what is growing seasonally, and to increase your exposure to the wide variety of fruits and vegetables. I have many clients that pick a vegetable they like, and eat it all the time because they have it classified as healthy, such as broccoli or kale. Too much of anything can lead to build up of metabolites, or habituation in the body. We need a complex array of vitamins and minerals and phytonutrients to thrive. The best way to assure this is to rotate the plants you are eating. My kids and I play a game where we pick five fruits and vegetables each week at the Farmers' Market, which we did not eat the week before. If we see something new—from cactus to sunchokes—we look up recipes and try them out.

You have to be vegetarian

Most people think that to be a good yogi or to live Ayurvedically, you have to be vegetarian. For me, listening to the energetics of your digestion, and matching its needs is Ayurvedic diet. Sometimes, your body may be asking for animal foods. Interestingly, there are specific times where Ayurveda advocates for animal foods, and these are usually states of deep depletion, for example, bone broths when fighting a cold. However, a plant-based diet is really ideal for nutrients, ease of digestion, and healthy energetics with our planet.

People often ask me if I'm a vegetarian. I'm not. I have been. But really, I'm not an anything-arian anymore. I'm simply committed to listening to what my body is asking for. If one day that is meat, or eggs, I'll partake; if it's not, I won't. I'd say I'm about 90 percent plant-based in what my body is naturally asking for, and most clients that are really listening to their bodies report majority plant-based diets.

If you are eating meat, I'd encourage you to not order it in restaurants that are using mass produced meat with chemicals and inhumane practices. Under the practice of *ahimsa*, we do want to ensure that any animal foods have been treated with love and respect for the nourishment they are providing us. We want to honor their lives and use all parts of their sacrifice for our benefit—similarly to how all hunting tribes from around the world operated—in reverence. Of course, in our lives, the closest we can get is free-range, grass-fed, happy animals. Our purchasing power will help to encourage this approach to the industry, so if you are going to partake in fish or meat, I encourage you to only choose restaurants and food products that engage in these practices.

With the fake or alternative meat industry on the rise, it's important to note that if these foods are heavily processed, with preservatives or GMO soy, they may not be better for your body, or easier to digest, than healthy meat.

You have to give up what you love to eat

When I first saw a Traditional Chinese Medicine practitioner, she made me give up my daily chai because the black tea and the warming chai spices (ginger, cardamom, black pepper) were too heating for me. I did it, and it helped, but I was also miserable and resentful towards her! Ayurveda taught me that there is always a way to substitute or modify to eat what you love. I developed a chai blend that used a less heating tea, and had a blend of spices and rose petals that was not heating, and supported my digestion and anxiety. Maybe you don't get down in the kitchen like that. You can still modify. Let's take toast as an example. Dry cold bread from the fridge placed in a toaster, ends up dessicated and crunchy and basically Vata. I could tell all people with Vata digestive features that they simply cannot eat toast. However, I'd rather think of a way to modify the qualities. If we take the same bread, and pan brown it in ample ghee or coconut oil with a bit of salt, or cinnamon, we've made it more warm, more moist, and spiced and more Vata balancing.

Healthy eating tips for everyone

As I mentioned earlier, our needs from food are changing and varied, and this makes static food rules not a great idea. However, there are some basic food principles that are great for everyone, all the time! If you're able to incorporate these balancing approaches to food, that's probably more significant than constantly modifying which *dosha* you're balancing.

Eat fresh

The fresher your food is—i.e. the shorter the time from harvest or slaughter to it being eaten—the more life force (*prana*) you will get from it. The whole purpose of eating is to gain life force, so this is important. This is also why Ayurveda does not advocate for making large batches of food that you keep reheating all week. In fact, refrigerating and reheating is viewed as a sort of processing of food, and contributes to toxic build-up. Maybe you don't have a lifestyle where you can cook fresh food each morning. Just start where you can. Throwing out food sooner, cooking a bit more often, letting leftovers come to room temperature naturally, not refrigerating what you can eat a few hours later, and eating at places that make food to order are all steps in the direction of increasing *prana*, and decreasing *ama*.

Eat wild

Wild food varieties have two to four times more phytonutrients than commercial varieties. In the supermarkets, we only see certain varieties, most of which are genetically modified. Phytonutrients are plant-based nutrients that do everything good in the body and fight against everything bad. I know that's a broad definition, but it's true. Wild means from your garden (started with organic heirloom seeds), or the Farmers' Market.

Cooking is an amazing form of self-care and loving

Everything you put into the food goes in the body, including love. You can taste it when food is made with love and care. For this reason, cooking can be a meditation, and we can infuse our food with loving intention. When food is prepared in hectic, stressful, mass-produced energetics, we take those in as well. In Ayurveda, we don't recommend cooking or eating when you are angry or sad, as these energetics will go into your tummy. My cousin's father-in-law has not ever eaten "out." The Indian man in his 90s has only eaten food cooked by his mother, his wife, and close family friends. When they travel, his wife cooks their food and peels fresh fruit for them to eat. I was so impressed with this level of awareness about the energetics he is taking in his body. Of course, they grow food and this is an extreme, yet inspiring, example. Just being aware of the energetics your food is being prepared with may, at the very least, help you shift where you choose to eat.

Many of us have a hard time nourishing ourselves. It's a byproduct of modern culture which teaches us that our value is in what we do, or produce, or accomplish. Starting to cook for yourself, however basic, is a great practice with which to begin a self-care lifestyle. I take time, and energy, to make good food for myself and this elevates my subconscious level of self-worth. Ultimately, prioritizing nourishing ourselves is an act of self-love. It's also a beautiful way to nourish and love those we cook for. It increases our union with our food, nature, our bodies—mindful union and presence is yoga.

Cooking is yoga.

Eat organic and non GMO

This one should be obvious, but it's not easy. Even in health food markets, most of the food is not organic, and a lot of food contains items such as soy, corn starch, corn syrup, and soy lecithin that are made from GMO soy and corn. It's impressive and scary how pervasive GMO foods are, and some estimates say 80–90 percent of "food" in conventional markets contain GMO ingredients. You'll have to read labels, and at this point, I'd assume all soy and corn related ingredients are GMO unless it specifically says "organic."

In the United States, pesticides which are known to be neurotoxic or carcinogenic are still in use, and the industry is poorly regulated. Most GMO foods have pesticide "partners" that they are marketed with to increase crop yields and profit margins. In the process, we are polluting the Earth, killing important insects, and ruining nature's balancing ecosystems. Not to mention that every inorganic pesticide is also poison for us humans. In India, depressed farmers who have had their land and crops devastated by GMO politics are committing suicide by drinking these poisonous pesticides.[1]

It's not easy to be 100 percent organic in modern urban settings, but it's more readily available day by day. Look for restaurants that offer local farm-fresh foods, and shop at the Farmers' Market—these are two easy ways to greatly increase your organic, non GMO food content, and to drive the market towards this healthier-for-all approach.

Honor your personal portion

If you cup your two hands together into the shape of a bowl, that's your personal portion size. Not a heaping bowl, but imagine filling your two hands with a level bowl. The "cupped hands" bowl approximates the size of your stomach, and is a good way to gauge an ideal personal portion. I recommend finding a bowl that matches this amount, and using it for a week. After you eat everything out of this one bowl, you'll train your eye to be able to see how much is a good amount of food for one sitting. While certain cultures seem well aware of this (French, Spanish, Japanese), others encourage over consumption (American). You can eat as often as you are hungry. However, the idea is that this amount is how much your stomach can handle in one sitting. If you are going to eat more, aka have dessert, then lengthening the total meal time helps to give time for your stomach to digest the extra amount (think of a long drawn out meal in Italy). Post-meal digestives are also helpful, such as an espresso, fennel seeds, digestive liquor, or herbal spice mix. Watching your personal portion helps greatly with not overburdening your *agni*, and preventing build-up.

Cleansing and fasting

No matter how much you try to match your food intake to your *agni*, we all are going to have some build-up over time. Various states of depletion, cravings, and default food choices happen. Ayurveda recommends cleansing each Spring and Fall as a basic lifestyle practice. There are many different ways to cleanse and detox, and exploring all the options and their various benefits and downfalls is beyond our scope here. What I

---

1   Sainath (2018). For links to more information and research, also see https://en.wikipedia. org/wiki/Farmers%27_suicides_in_India

will suggest is that you start to listen to when you have the natural urge or inspiration to cleanse.

Kitchardi (Mung stew) cleansing has become popular in the yoga community, and it's relatively safe and easy. Intermittent fasting and juice cleanses are also easy. Activated charcoal and teas to flush the liver are also simple and readily available. What kind of cleansing you do, when, and how, and how long, will all depend on your Current State and the energetics of your life at that time. More extreme cleanses, such as the famous "Master Cleanse" may actually be okay during the damp heaviness of the Spring, whereas they would be too depleting for the Fall/ Winter. Warm kitchardi cleansing would be a better fit for the Vata at the end of the year, or the Vata of your life if you don't have the ability to be still and unscheduled while cleansing. A green juice cleanse would be best during the high Pitta of the summer because it's so cooling. Cleansing can be as simple or complex as you make it. I have a friend that does one day of liquid nourishment each week, and that's her way of giving her digestive system a regular break from having to work hard. You could do a three-week long intensive *Pancha Karma* cleanse in India too, and that would be more involved with specific foods, herbs, routines, and body therapeutics. For our purposes, being aware of the need to cleanse at least once or twice a year at the bare minimum, and learning how to avoid too much, or too rich, foods on occasion is sufficient.

Summary

Balancing digestion is like riding a unicorn. Even still, there is so much you can do to take significant steps towards being more in tune with your body and its needs with food and eating. In summary:

- Cultivate connection to appetite, and thus digestive capacity.

- Cultivate connection to food, and the qualities/*doshas* you are taking in.

- Shift to healthier eating habits first.

- Cleanse and fast periodically.

The bidirectional relationship
between digestion and emotion

Earlier, I presented pathogenesis progression from subtle energetic body to the physical. This presents a more linear initial formation of an imbalance. While the majority of imbalance starts out this way, an imbalanced body also affects how we feel. When the body is not optimal, it, in turn, creates disturbances in the mind and emotions. The Western exploration on the gut-brain connection is a great example of how the physical microbiome affects the mind and emotions. Menopause is another one in which physical hormone levels modulate emotional states. Lack of sleep, low blood sugar, shortness of breath, and even orgasm are other examples of the physical affecting the emotional. This highlights the importance of supporting *all parts of ourselves.*

Chapter 9

EMOTIONAL WELLNESS

How to Understand and Address Your Emotional Experience

Learning objectives

- Get a sense of how Ayurveda views emotional wellness.

- Learn a basic framework to interpret your feelings.

- Get a sense of how to approach balance for the emotional body.

There are millions of books on shaping your mental and emotional landscape. Here, we'll focus on some basics for emotional wellness adapted from Ayurveda. These tools and approaches are both acute and accumulative in their benefits, so the more you apply them, the more benefit you'll feel. Time and practice will allow emotional wellness to blossom, but again, it's not linear.

Just as I've been weaving emotional awareness through this book, emotional wellness is woven through every aspect of our life experience. To give steps to emotional wellness is a ridiculous concept; yet, how else do we begin to learn things other than to have them simplified and structured? The limitations of oversimplified approaches apply here, although our goal is to increase your awareness and understanding of your emotional experience. We'll begin with a bit of an overview of feelings, and what psychospiritual wellness could look like. Then, we'll go into some tools to begin your balancing practice.

Psychospiritual wellness

What is "psychospiritual wellness"?

I like to define "psychospiritual" as everything beyond the physical body: emotions, mindset, attitude, aura, vibrational frequency, spirit, soul, intuition, etc. I'll use the terms emotional body and subtle energetic body interchangeably here.

I purposely include "spiritual" when discussing Ayurvedic psychology, because spiritual growth is like the blossom on the tree of emotional wellness. A healthy tree produces plentiful beautiful blossoms. Said more plainly, you cannot have spiritual growth without moments of emotional harmony; applying your emotional awareness towards more harmonious choices *is* spiritual growth. The more whole, happy, and connected you feel, the more your awareness grows, and the more you choose "whole, happy, and connected" experiences—from food to relationships. The more you have these "whole, happy,and connected" experiences, the more whole, happy, and connected your spirit feels.

Beyond therapy

I also use the term "psychospiritual" to convey the distinction from Western psychology—in which spirituality has been rinsed out. Coming from a neuroscience and psychiatry background, I felt like Ayurveda gave me the missing piece in emotional wellness—*how to receive and respond to my own emotional body in the moment.* This is a big deal. Nothing can replace our inner guidance—no therapist, no research, no guru, no motivational speaker on YouTube.

In the West, we're suffering from the same patriarchal overlays in psychology that we have in medicine. We outsource the interpretation of our emotional states to therapists. Our tools in psychology and psychiatry are limited. We can analyze the past, and come to greater understanding of why certain patterns exist in our emotional experience. We can even increase our awareness of our emotional and functional responses to certain events to shift outcomes. But that's really it, and the limitations are why we lean towards medicating so heavily. Therapy can be insight-generating and supportive, especially when it includes processes and tools that put you in the driver's seat of shifting your patterns.

Without the ability to interpret our own emotional experiences, and respond in real time, we remain dependent on the practitioner of emotional wellness. More importantly, we may miss the opportunity to hear our own emotional feedback on our life choices. This leads us to engage in situations in which our emotional needs are unmet, or in which we have internal conflict. We choose these situations for all the reasons in our minds that we've been programmed to prioritize from our culture, family, generation. In trying to do *what we think we should*, we override the emotional signals, and this will lead to emotional suffering every time we do it.

Mind and emotional body as partners

In Ayurveda, we honor the emotional system and the mind as partners in aligned decision making. In other words, you want to feel great, and think well, about your choices. You cannot find this alignment if you're not listening to your emotions. When you do, your feelings can help you figure out how to choose anything. In the last chapter, I had you check in with your digestive system about what would feel really good to eat. Similarly, we can use emotional feedback to guide any other decision, what to wear to whom to sleep with. To not use one entire system would be like running with one leg. It's more like awkwardly hopping through life when you only utilize your mental ability.

Reshaping your thoughts, emotions, and experience

Of course, with imprinting from our life experience, we often believe that what would feel best is unavailable to us—from a great partner to abundance to a job we love. It may take years of thought repatterning to strip away those limiting belief systems. It's a lifelong practice.

> Neuroplasticity, the notion that our experiences and perceptions affect the brain's functioning and structure, is a relatively new discovery, but it matches what sages have known for millennia about how the mind shapes the physical world, including the brain.[1]

Although we are not all created equally, we do all have equal potential to manifest any desired emotional experience in Ayurveda. In fact, each of the *doshas* provides its own benefits towards manifesting your desired experience: Vata allows us to imagine what could be, to be richly

---

1   Villoldo (2015, p.29)

inspired, and visualize well. Pitta gives us clarity on what we seek, and discernment to choose accordingly. Kapha allows the fertile, dreamy and peaceful receptivity to attract our desired experience.

Vedic psychospiritual principles consider all aspects of our human experience. We look at the patterns in what we experience and what we choose. As I mentioned in the beginning of the book, this is an empowerment based practice, in which *we choose* the energetics of our life experience. As we become more aware of perspectives and thought response patterns in our minds, we combine that information with the report from the emotional body on how those patterns *feel*. The emotional feedback and the mental analysis, together, let us know if the pattern is serving us, or if we need to respond differently. By choosing differently, we create experiences different from our previous imprints and beliefs, and reshape our life experiences.

What emotional wellness could feel like

Ayurveda observes the patterns from the perspectives of the *doshas*, our emotional needs, internal conflict, interconnection, and life purpose. In other words, we're taking a spherical view of your emotional experience. Ideally, we then apply this awareness towards choosing patterns that are a better energetic fit, and get positive feedback from the emotional body. In this way, Ayurveda incorporates the psychodynamic approach of pattern identification (causes and effects), and the cognitive behaviorial approach of shifting responses, and takes emotional wellness several steps beyond that.

I'll define emotional wellness as feeling open, free of internal conflict, empowered in meeting our own emotional needs, connected to our inner guidance, loved and comfortable in our relations, on our life paths, and ever increasing in our consciousness of the energetics we are choosing. This definition of emotional wellness acknowledges that we are more than physical beings, and that our life experience is one we can modulate.

AYURVEDA
AND PSYCHOLOGY

PSYCHODYNAMIC	COGNITIVE BEHAVIORAL	AYURVEDA
Discovering why the patterns are what they are	Traits and practices of happiness	What is my nature and how does that affect my decision making?
	Adjusting behavioral responses	What are my deeper emotional needs and how do I show up for them?
	$E + R = O$	
		How can I resolve my internal conflicts?
		Am I on my path?

Figure 9.1 *Western and Ayurvedic considerations in psychology*

Feelings and emotional needs

Just as your circulatory system affects every part of your body, so too does your emotional body. The emotional body communicates to the mind via feelings. The brain, heart, glandular and nervous systems coordinate a neurobiophysiological response to each one of our feelings, which then affects every tissue system.

Controlling and coping

Modern life is one big practice of turning off your feelings, or trying to control them. In the West, we treat our emotions like random good and bad experiences. Unpleasant emotions are categorized as "bad" and we're encouraged to do whatever it takes to just stop feeling that way. This victimized approach to unpleasant feelings plays into the rise of common coping responses, like suicide, Netflix binging, porn addiction, antidepressants, or even yoga retreats. We do so many things to escape feeling bad, and most are temporary band-aids. Even meditation can be a short-term coping response to alleviate the distress of unpleasant feelings. Neither medication or "primordial sound" meditation is really getting to the root cause of that feeling. We want to be able to understand why it is we have the feelings we do.

Feelings messages

Feelings are functional feedback from the emotional body, just like poop is from the digestive body. The quality of stool is how digestion communicates that something needs to be adjusted or not. When I have loose stools (P symptom), I become aware that my choices have caused imbalance in my digestive system, and I adjust my food choices accordingly. When I have constipation (V symptom), I know I need to adjust again, and in a different way than when I have loose stools. If the adjustments I'm making are working, my digestive system will communicate that with nice healthy bowel movements. Each poop is a message—an informative alert, or a validation that choices are energetically balanced. I don't want to have a lifelong dependence on laxatives, or anti-diarrheal medication, as I'd be missing the message, and the information on how to adjust. Instead, I want to change my eating to make the balancing shifts, and see in my poop that pattern is successfully shifted. In other words, I want to hear the alerts and use the information to address the root cause, until I get a validation message that my efforts are working.

Feelings are functional.

Similarly, each feeling is a message—an informative alert, or a validation. As I mentioned earlier, feelings are how our emotional bodies communicate with our minds. Pleasant emotions are encouragement from the emotional body that we are choosing in a way that feels good to our inner psyche and subtle energetics. Unpleasant emotions are messages that we're choosing in a way that doesn't feel good. They are a message to reflect and consider what is disharmonious in the energetics of our lives. Just as the symptom (loose stools or constipation) disappears when we meet the needs of the digestive body, so too does the unpleasant emotion when we meet the needs of the emotional body. When emotional needs are met, unpleasant feelings dissipate—they are no longer needed as alert messages. When we learn how to hear and respond to our feelings, we can receive the powerful guidance from our emotional body.

The "Psychospiritual Spiral"

Of course, changing how we eat is a lot simpler in many ways than changing how we choose the energetics of everything that affects the emotional body. Additionally, life will keep bringing opportunities to feel stress or conflict. It's a cyclical journey—unpleasant feelings lead to increased awareness, leads to changed perspectives and responses, lead to pleasant feelings, lead to less active attention on choices, leads to imbalancing choices, lead to unpleasant feelings. And around again. I call this the Psychospiritual Spiral, and while we cannot change the cyclical emotional experience, we can change the amount of time we spend in the feel-good part of our experience. And that's our goal—to spend as much of our lives in the top arc of this cycle. There are many ways, and tools, to support that goal.

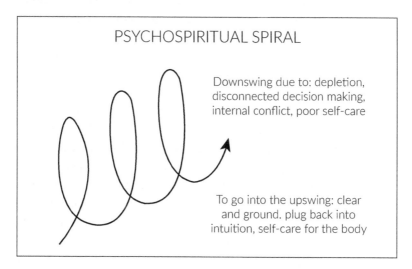

Figure 9.2 *The Psychospiritual Spiral of our emotional experience*

The balancing approach below is comprised of what seems most effective, and universal, based on my 10 years of exploring this topic personally and professionally. I've distilled down to create a clear, doable process which you can use every time you find yourself on the downward arc. How do you know if you're on the downward arc? You feel unpleasant feelings, heavily and frequently. Which unpleasant feelings are there will vary with Current State, karmic lessons, and Constitutional tendencies and for this reason, getting too caught up in breaking down the details of the unpleasant feelings isn't worthwhile. Instead we'll focus on getting to the root cause of feelings, and supporting our emotional body as its needs are being met.

Step 1. Identify your feelings and unmet emotional needs.

Step 2. Balance the *doshas*, and take care of the basics to feel good.

Step 3. Practice feeling how you would if the emotional needs were met.

Balancing approach

Step 1. Identify your feelings and unmet emotional needs

Identify feelings for the sake of acknowledging and accepting where you are emotionally. Then, shift your focus to the message of the emotion—unpleasant feelings reveal unmet emotional needs. Emotional needs can seem vague and abstract, but they are simple and intuitive. Your emotional needs are what you need to feel better, or relieved. Despite the fact that we don't always take the time to consider our emotional needs, most can express what would feel better, in any circumstance.

Discover emotional needs by asking, "What would feel really good in this situation?" The answer to that question typically unveils the emotional need. Let's say I'm feeling anxious, and my answer of what would feel better is, " I just wanna know it's gonna be okay; and I don't want to care so much that I get like this; and I think a few nights of good sleep would help me feel better." Reassurance, decreased attachment to outcome, and sleep would all be my emotional needs in this example (and in this lifetime).

Maybe I'm only able to identify two of the needs (reassurance and sleep) on my own, and my mentor helped me see the need for the third. It doesn't matter. There are usually multiple emotional needs in any situation, and in this case, there could be a fourth and fifth uncovered later. We may only be aware of some in the beginning, and learn of other unmet needs in time. Just start with trying to meet the needs you are aware of and can meet most easily and you'll be heading in the right direction. In the present example, this could look like a few days of prioritizing plentiful and deep sleep. Maybe next, I start meeting my need for reassurance by chanting (Bijas for the *Muladhara* and *Anahata chakras*), and listening to guided meditations that help me feel more like everything is okay. Being able to meet your own needs is powerful medicine for low self worth, and fear and worry.

AWARENESS BEFORE ACTION

Our whole perspective on our lives is based on how we feel about our life experience. To achieve a life in which you feel peaceful, with your emotional needs met, you need to feel this way in the micro decisions that make up this life. By regularly taking actions, decisions, expressions that forward your emotional wellness, you achieve internal harmony.

Take action *after* you've identified your emotional needs. In the beginning, you'll continue to act based on external needs. This is due to imprinted defaults and social conditioning, and it's normal. There's a big rewiring of how you approach decisions happening. It takes time and practice. Taking the time to consider how you may meet your emotional needs in the situation is a big first step. Next steps include choices that are partly meeting external and partly internal needs. Eventually, the needs for internal harmony are the focus of your choices.

Taking action before identifying your emotional needs in any situation is like driving left or right simply based on what traffic signals are in front of you, without ever identifying the destination.

LISTEN TO YOUR INTUITION

You know what would feel best to you deep down, and only you do. Just accept the first answers that come to mind when you ask yourself, "What would make me feel good, better, easier, relieved in this situation?" Even if you don't know how to meet your emotional needs at first, asking yourself this question regularly will help you become more in touch with what makes you feel best. That's organically going to shift your awareness.

Try to find at least three emotional needs every time you practice this self-reflective exercise. It helps you to get out of a linear cause-effect framework, and gets you in the habit of recognizing the many emotional needs you have.

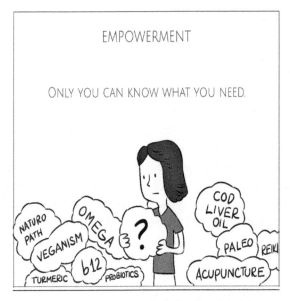

Figure 9.3 *Empowerment in feeling based decisions*

Step 2. Balance the **doshas,** *and take care of the basics to feel good*

Meeting your emotional needs may take some time. In the meantime, balance the *doshas* in your life. Take a look at your *Signs of Imbalance Chart* and/or your *Current State Survey* (Appendix 4). What *doshas* are revealed in your present feeling states? Bring in opposite qualities in as many ways as you can think of, as we walked through in Chapter 6.

It's more direct to shift the energetics in your mind, as mind-states and feeling states go hand-in-hand. *Pranayama* and chanting have the most direct influence on our mind-state because of the way the breath, sounds, and thought systems and energetic channels (*srotas*) are interconnected.

Chanting

Chanting Hindu Sanskrit *mantras* isn't for everyone. However, seed sounds, or *Bija Mantras*, are effective and easy to use because they are so short and easy to pronounce. Each *Bija Mantras* balances specific *chakras*, and specific emotional and physical functions. In Chart 9.1, the emotional balancing effects of *Bija Mantras* are listed by *dosha*.

Chart 9.1 *Bija Mantras* for Emotional Balancing

V	P	K
Balancing Effects of *Bija Mantras*		
Lum—increased stability decreased fear Vum—increased creative potency Rum—improved understanding and solving Yum—increased self-love Kshum—increased clarity Om—harmonizing; homeostasis	Vum—increased creative potency Yum—decreased intensity and overanalysis Kshum—balanced perception, prevent righteousness Om—harmonizing; homeostasis	Rum—improved understanding and solving Yum—decreased emotional baggage Hum—increased expression Kshum—increased clarity Om—harmonizing; homeostasis

FEEL GOOD FIRST

We'll cover balancing *doshas* with *Pranayama, asana,* music, and aromatherapy—all powerful ways to affect mind-state, in the next chapter. In the meantime, get your basics in place—good food, good sleep, self-care (see Chapter 6).

All acts of self-care and nourishment help to move us up out of the downward arc of the Psychospiritual Spiral. Once we are feeling more rejuvenated, we're going to find solutions and clarity that we cannot access from a place of internal discord and depletion. For this reason, focus on feeling better *before* you solve anything else. It's like giving a plant consistent water, sun, and love before you get into solving a micronutrient analysis of the soil.

Step 3. Practice feeling how you would if the emotional needs were met

Most everything we desire is to have a feeling experience, to meet an emotional need. I crave a hot mug of chai to feel calm, warmed, and grounded; a speaking gig to feel successful, worthy, impactful; a tropical climate to feel supple and relaxed. We seek people, places, things, and experiences based on *our ideas* of what those energetics would feel like. Along the way, we get attached to the people, places, things, and experiences, and forget to evaluate how these energetic inputs feel.

Oftentimes, what we think something is going to feel like doesn't match our experience. The cup of chai could be consumed mindlessly while cleaning the house. It wasn't savored, ended up getting cold, and the experience of the chai didn't result in feeling calm, warmed, or grounded. Similarly, the speaking gig could be an experience that felt anything but successful, worthy, or impactful. It happens all the time that our ideas, of what feelings people, places, things, and experiences will bring us, are off. They are mixed up with projection, fears, hopes, denial, imprints, past lives, karma, and more.

While no person, place, thing, or experience guarantees the desired feeling, practicing feeling that way does. Let's say we have a woman who is depressed and anxious, and realizes a common emotional need across many areas of her life is to feel worthy (acknowledged, deserving). She consciously practices feeling worthy, starting by journaling about what makes her feel worthy. Soon, she starts noticing more when when she does and doesn't feel worthy, what factors affect her worthiness most directly, how others embody worthiness. She starts to make choices from a place of "What would the worthy version of me do? If I really felt worthy, how would I respond?" She becomes familiar with what worthy feels like, and what choices align with worthiness. Slowly, a few more minutes each day, she's feeling, and witnessing feeling, worthy. With changed perception and emotional response to life situations, cellular environment are changed. She's feeling more worthy because she chose to, and her physiologic response to that feeling benefits her body.

This sounds easier than it is because this practice also requires that any time you feel opposite to your desired feelings, you stop and change. With the above example, the practice would include not speaking, acting, or thinking in ways that didn't allow her to feel worthy. It requires paying attention, and bravely choosing different words, actions, and thoughts.

She applied her awareness (to choose worthiness), and this means she was in a process of spiritual growth. That she did start to feel more worthy is confirmation that her choices were indeed being made from a place which best served her emotional wellbeing. In response to feeling unworthy, she consciously evolved her way of operating to shift her experience. This is deliberate psychospiritual growth, and inextricable from emotional wellness in Ayurveda.

Summary

- Emotional wellness includes psychospiritual considerations and is a cyclical experience.

- Feelings are functional messages from the emotional body, revealing unmet emotional needs.

- Emotional wellness is a powerful way to support the physical body and prevent disease, and vice versa.

- Healing is a process of spiritual growth: increased awareness fueling new choices.

- Practicing feeling your desired emotions is the only guaranteed way to feel them more.

Chapter 10

AYURVEDA IN LEADING YOGA

Modifying Energetics in Yoga

Learning objectives

- Understand the importance of personal experience with Ayurveda.

- Begin to consider the doshic effects of *asana*.

- Get a sense of ways to modulate energetics in your instruction, and the space.

- Have a starting place for modifying approaches in group and private settings.

The importance of personal experience

Could you imagine leading someone in "downdog" without ever having practiced the pose yourself? Let's say you read all about it, looked at pictures, and tried to teach the pose. There would be something huge missing—your experience—with it, in it, in the various ways that your body has shown up for it over time; the ways you've had to adjust, what you've realized, how you've modified, what hurt, what felt good. Your experience is what makes the pose come alive in your instruction, and become more relatable and accessible to your students.

It's the same with Ayurveda, and anything really. In the West, we reduce down everything and try to promise incredible results in the shortest amount of time. Incredible results come from *more* time, consistency, and depth of experience. There's that saying that a little knowledge can be a dangerous thing, and I think that's because a small slice of any body of wisdom can be shifted dramatically depending on what context you put around it. This is why really getting to know the entire context is helpful. You get "downdog" more when you understand the context of balancing effort and ease, of lengthening the spine, of engaging *tribandha*. If you didn't have this greater context, you may instruct the pose in a way that misses its benefits, or worse, causes harm. As you add more context around "downdog"—awareness of the weight distribution in the hands, the spiraling rotation of the muscles around the arm and leg bones, and the *Yamas*—the pose becomes a richer experience, and has more benefits to more parts of you.

This has been the aim of the book so far, to give you as much insight as possible to bring Ayurveda in your life, so you can begin to experience it. Just like anything else in life, experience creates the foundation to be able to "Walk the talk." Like yoga, it's only through your personal experience of Ayurveda that you will bring it to life for others. This is why the starting place for you to interweave Ayurveda into your teaching is for you to interweave it in your own life. Once you start seeing the patterns all around you, and the *doshas* dancing within them, you won't be able to turn off that awareness. That's the place from which to organically, effortlessly, offer it as a part of your yoga teaching. Give yourself as long as you need to *feel the doshas*, and then bring it in your teaching. Even if you never bring it in your teaching, but can have preliminary insights in your own physical and emotional balancing shifts, that's still amazing and worthwhile.

Experience Ayurveda (before you teach it).

Ayurveda is based upon the principle of Self-knowledge. Its goal is not simply health as an end in itself, but health as a basis for self-understanding, for the recognition of our true nature and living in accord with it. [Thus,] Ayurveda naturally directs us towards the path of Yoga... Ayurveda thus always aims at self-care, teaching the individual how to live in harmony with his or her own nature... For this reason, the educational part of Ayurveda is perhaps more important than the treatment side. Its self-care approach is perhaps more important than its clinical approach. It is not enough that we as practitioners or healers know certain things about ... how to improve their condition.

What matters is that they know these things and learn how to apply the tools for themselves that will change their condition.[1]

As expressed in the quote above, the spirit of Ayurveda is an empowered one. At its core is the constant teaching and uplifting of ourselves, and one another. We're not really practicing Ayurveda by asking people to take a "*dosha* quiz" or telling them not to eat salad in the winter. As with Yoga, so too with Ayurveda do we want to encourage our students to examine their patterns and increase their self awareness.

To this end, teach *why* when you bring in recommendations based on Ayurvedic awareness. When you have students flex the foot in a pose, and you tell them that it serves to protect the knee, they'll know apply that adjustment on their own whenever they want to stabilize the knee. Similarly, we want to provide the basis for the recommendations based in Ayurveda. Keeping in touch with "the why" behind balancing choices ensures they don't become rote rules.

In sharing the nuances of your personal experience with Ayurvedic awareness and shifts you'll have greater positive impact. You're an example of someone a few steps ahead on a lifestyle path that they are interested in, and students always appreciate hearing your journey and relating to someone who is heading in the same direction. My hope is that you'll not only inspire them to learn more about Ayurveda, but to do so in an awareness-increasing manner.

Doshas in *asana*

You may have heard "yoga for your *dosha*" and other such attempts to have you type yourself and then practice certain poses based on your "*dosha* type." While an unchanging, Constitution-based approach is bit silly, it's nice to consider the energetics of *asana*. Each pose has specific effects on the physical body—which muscles it lengthens, or strengthens, for example. Additionally, each pose has inherent ability to shift *doshas*.

In general, poses are considered balancing for *doshas* if they counteract the symptoms of imbalance for that *dosha*. For example, Vata imbalance commonly involves overstimulation, gas and constipation, and lower back weakness. Thus, forward folding poses decrease Vata, as they represent a coming into yourself, and help to remove gas in the lower abdomen. Similarly, *trikonasana* would be Vata balancing because it strengthens

---

1   Frawley (2006, p.121)

the low back and engages the lower abdomen. Seated and floor poses are grounding, and thus balancing for Vata's light, airy qualities.

Pitta imbalance tends to involve excess heat in the Pitta digestive organs. Thus, backbends help to balance Pitta, as do twists and backbends which tone the liver, spleen, and small intestines. Pitta imbalance also commonly involves a lot of tension in the neck, shoulders, jaw, and forehead. So any poses which stretch and help to release tension in these areas would be Pitta balancing.

Kapha balancing poses would counteract the Kapha tendency to be still, heavy, stagnant. So poses which are heating and stimulate circulation of blood and lymphatics would be a good fit. Kapha tends to accumulate in the chest, so heart openers and backbends balance this Kapha tendency.

All of the above examples are generalizations based on the physical functionality of a pose. Another way to assess the energetic effects of a pose is to *feel* what qualities are experienced. This will be more accurate because it's based on *what you sense* than what you think. For example, the "Warrior poses" will traditionally increase qualities such as warm, strong, focused, active, and aligned. These qualities will increase P, but are opposite to and will thus decrease Vata and Kapha.

However, all qualities can be shifted based on how the pose is practiced. Let's say you're in "Warrior 1" for a quick moment in the middle of a vinyasa flow class. You're unlikely to ground in it, or receive the traditional qualities of the pose. It's too momentary. The main qualities may be "moving, fast," and maybe there's compression in the low back from over-arching without a solidly established base. In this example, the experience of "Warrior 1" has qualities which increase Vata, don't do much for Pitta, and decrease Kapha.

Chart 10.1 Examples of VPK balancing qualities in *asana* categories and yoga styles

Dosha	Vata balancing	Pitta balancing	Kapha balancing
Asana types	Forward folds	Twists	Inversions
	Seated poses	Prone poses	Standing poses
	Supine poses	Supine poses	Balancing poses
	Standing poses	Passive supported poses	Warrior poses
	Warrior poses	Digestive poses	Core-strengthening poses
	Core-strengthening poses	Hip openers	Heart openers
	Balancing poses	Neck and shoulder openers	

Yoga styles	Yin	Yin	Dynamic movements in poses
	Core Power	Gentle	Vinyasa
	Bikram	Slow Flow	Viniyoga
	Heated	Hatha	Bikram
	Ashtanga		Hatha
	Hatha		

These theoretical energetics of a pose are more felt when we are practicing classic *asana* alone, present for five or more breaths long. This is more the vibe of a home practice. When you start your practice of tapping into what qualities/*doshas* you feel in various poses, you'll notice is that the qualities you experience change depending on how you practice them. Just like food (think of the cabbage and the toast examples in Chapter 8: Digestive Wellness), the energetics of *asana* are modifiable.

Sivasana is traditionally a relaxing pose (effect: decrease V, decrease P, increase K). If I cue with "Tuck the chin to elongate the neck along the floor. In fact, try to get the entire length of the spine in contact with the ground beneath you. Widen the upper back and separate the shoulder blades. Anchor the shoulders to the ground. As you find additional length in the spine, shift the pelvis down a bit. Ensure your arms and legs are symmetrical." These cues make the pose active, turn on the mind, and encourage analysis and adjustment—all qualities that increase Pitta, and decrease the traditionally passive relaxed qualities we associate with *Sivasana*. If I rattle off these cues quickly, students may feel a bit like they didn't catch everything, and may be a bit caught off guard with having any instruction in *Sivasana* and these qualities would increase Vata in their experience of the pose. All of the qualities in the example above would decrease the pose's balancing effects for P and V.

Let's say I'm instructing Warrior 2, but in a way that doesn't emphasize traditional Pitta qualities. "Feel the Earth beneath your feet, and shift back and forth until your hips organically find a middle balance between your front and back legs. Open the palms to the sky, and face forward, opening the heart and collar bones while elongating the neck. Close your eyes, and feel supported by the ground. Allow the hips to feel heavy and draw the tailbone down towards the Earth. With every inhale, expand the front of the chest, and feel open. With every exhale, release tension in the shoulders and hips and feel grounded." I've shifted the qualities to be more grounding, opening, centered, and relaxed. It's no longer with the intensity and *dhristi*, and active nature. This shift in how I instruct changed the energetics of the pose to be a lot less Pitta. The grounding and eyes closed approach are balancing for Vata. The opening across the front of the chest is balancing for Kapha, as is the active stance in the limbs. Closing the eyes, making the post more feeling-based, and removing the turn of the neck are all modifications that balance Pitta. So, I've ended up with a pose that has qualities and aspects that balance all three *doshas*.

You can use this awareness in planning the energetics of your class. But you can also use these shifts in qualities to give individual modifications. Once you get beyond planning, and have the more intuitive teaching style of advanced teachers, you can tailor energetics to the students' needs in real time. Some teachers check in with students beforehand on injuries and what they are feeling that day, and I highly recommend this if you are comfortable enough to shift energetics "on the fly."

With these two examples, you can see how the traditional qualities of a pose are easily shifted based on how you cue and modify. In addition to how you instruct, the major shifter of energetics of the pose is you. Your vibe that day, your Current State, your presence, your voice, your movement around the room, etc. We've all experienced how the energetics we're feeling that day can affect the way we teach, and how we hold space as instructors. You can sense when a teacher comes in the room and they're grounded, and there for you, or when they're caught up in studio politics or selling services. Being aware of the energetics our students are feeling from us also helps us feel more interconnected and humble.

The energetics of your teaching

Hopefully, you're already trying to be more in touch with your Current State, bringing in some initial balancing shifts, and doing your best to support your being in a good feeling place to teach. Let's review some of the major ways to shift the energetics of a pose that you can plan for.

Speech

A large part of leading yoga is instructing with your voice. Although we have our natural cadence and tone, we can be aware of the qualities of our speech as qualities that our students are absorbing for the hour or so that they are with us. Within the category of speech, we can consider pace, tone, and emotional valence as significant ways to shift qualities. Slowing down the speed of your instruction will decrease Vata, and allows students to digest your instruction more easefully. Quicker pace will increase Vata (speed) and Pitta (rate of hearing and responding) and students will report feeling more anxious (V) about keeping up, and more in their minds (P). Lower tones and deeper pitches increase K qualities, while higher pitch and louder instruction (think military style) would increase P (intense) and V (stimulating) qualities. If I have a light, happy, easy-go-lucky emotional state, you will hear that in my speech. Consider the contrast if I'm with an expert, no fluff, serious approach. It's great to examine how you want your students to feel, and to match the emotional undertone of your speech, and which words you choose.

Sequencing

While sequencing is a broad term, consider how you order the poses, how long in the pose, and the qualities of the transitions. Let's take a Bikram sequence as a example. It's very Pitta in its qualities. There is a specific order to the poses that is considered optimal, the timing is strict, and about 95 percent of the entire sequence is active. There is no relaxing into any poses. It's constant attention, effort, and analysis throughout the sequence, and the length of the poses encourages active progress. The heat, the mirrors to encourage optimal form, and the instructors correcting you are additional P qualities in Bikram. By contrast, a yin sequence may have far fewer poses, held for much longer but passively so. These qualities decrease V, decrease P, and increase K. In a Yin approach, we'll gently warm up the body first, and then come into deeper releasing poses. This approach is V reducing—warming, and then deep, still, and supported (with props). Obviously, Yin practice is great for balancing V, but Bikram practice is as well. The Yin sequence balances the excessive extroversion, stimulation, movement, and rigidity (myofascial) of Vata. Bikram's heat, structured and unchanging approach, and emphasis on clearly defined goals all balance Vata's unfocused, erratic, changing qualities. While Bikram's heating qualities and intense sequence are balancing for Kapha, the Yin sequence would not be. Conversely, the Yin sequence is balancing for Pitta (passive, release of control, and active doing), and Bikram sequence is not.

In general, spending more time in a pose allows for greater adjustment and strength building (P), or more time to release tension and stretch

(K; think of a passive seated forward fold *paschimotanasana*). It just depends how you cue and modify. Shorter poses and quicker transitions bring in more Vata. Core strength requiring transitions (e.g. Warrior 1 to stork pose) are more P building, while loosely defined (e.g. "slowly make your way to a seated position") transitions are more V. Transitions that are slow, on the ground, and easy have more K qualities.

Breathwork

How you direct students to breathe will shift the energetics of each pose. Having them do "breath of fire" *kapalabhati* breathing will increase Pitta even in a relaxed seated pose. So will Solar (right nostril) breathing, but you'll feel that it's less Pitta qualities than *kapalabhati*, and thus less heating in effect. *Sitali pranayama* (cooling breath) will help reduce Pitta in any pose, as will Lunar (left nostril) breathing. Audible exhales through the mouth will help to release muscle tension (reduce V and P) in any pose.

Having them slow down the breath cycle, and match the length of inhales and exhales, will greatly reduce Vata in any pose. The practice of drawing the attention to the breath is one of decreasing distraction and increasing connection of the mind and body, so most breathwork is Vata reducing. However, if the exhales are longer than the inhales, such as in *Bhastrika*, this can lead to hyperventilation and increased Vata. Those with Vata imbalance often feel really lightheaded immediately and may even pass out with breathing that increases Vata. Since most people have some degree of Vata imbalance ensuring that your breathing instruction isn't too Vata increasing is a good idea.

Where you direct focus

There are many Yoga Teacher Trainings which heavily emphasize an anatomical focus (e.g. "rotate the inner thigh externally") as part of practicing "correctly." It's great to have this knowledge of how to instruct anatomical cues and physical alignment based instruction to prevent injury. This approach is all P in quality (strict, analysis, correction). In contrast, feeling based cues (e.g. "feel as though the weight distribution between your hands and feet is even") are a lot more K in quality. Feeling based instruction is reducing for V and P, as it encourages getting out of the mind and being present with feeling, and isn't encouraging the student to meet some "to do" in a pose. Not directing the focus anywhere in a pose, as tends to happen in gym yoga, would be more Vata, as it leaves the focus to wander.

The imagery you bring in is a wonderful way to shift qualities of focus. I once had a teacher that taught in a way that I dubbed "Wu-Tang Yoga" as he would give us all this Shaolin warrior imagery while in poses: "See through the wall, beyond your opponent; Feel the energy extending from your fingertips through your opponent." This imagery increased Pitta qualities, and sure enough, I felt more confident and intense. I've had other teachers that used more Earth-based imagery (e.g. "allow your heart to melt towards the Earth"), and felt more grounded and self-loving (K) after an hour of receiving those images. During one yoga class I had a teacher that had an ecstatic dance session in the middle. To cue the dance, she encouraged us to embody all kinds of Vata imagery (wild, flowing, erratic, unpatterned, spontaneous), and the room instantly felt very Vata with the energetics of the movement and the instruction. The energetic qualities of the images you use infuse your instruction.

Chart 10.2 Examples of VPK balancing shifts in qualities of instruction

Qualities for...	Vata balancing	Pitta balancing	Kapha balancing
Speech	Slow Medium volume Less wordy Simple Calm	Slow Low volume Calm Accepting	Medium pace Medium to louder volume Inspiring Enthusiastic
Sequencing	Structured Same Slow paced Core strengthening Simple sequences that are easy to follow	Encourage modifications to meet your own best feel Slow build-up and wind down Longer, creative sequences they can't predict	Quicker pace Changing Core-strengthening, but not too challenging Dynamic movement Lots of short rest breaks
Breathwork	*Bhramari* *Anulom-Vilom/* *Nadi Shodana* *Ujjai*	Lunar Breathing Lion's Breath *Sitali*	Solar Breathing *Kapalabhati* *Bhastrika*
Focus	Breath focus Anatomical Gaze towards the ground *Dhristi/* focused gaze straight ahead	Feeling based Soft gaze or eyes closed Gaze towards the ground	Anatomical Strengthening Focused gaze straight ahead Upwards gaze Eyes open

In the illustration in Figure 10.1, the broader spheres indicate broader energetic influence on the student. You can see that all of the above aspects of how you instruct ("How you teach") combine with what you instruct ("*asana*") to have a great influence on the qualities the student takes in.

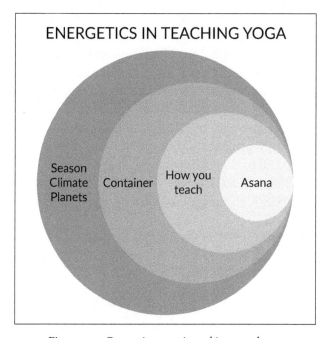

ENERGETICS IN TEACHING YOGA

Season Climate Planets   Container   How you teach   Asana

Figure 10.1 *Energetics experienced in yoga classes*

The "Container" includes all of the energetics of the place of practice. The energetics of "How you teach" forms the a significant portion of the energetics of the "Container" that the student is practicing in. In addition, we can observe the *doshas* in other aspects of the Container.

The energetics of the "Container"

Vaastu, and its more popular derivative, Feng-Shui, are sciences that examine the energetics of a given space. Here we are simply acknowledging the basics of what qualities the student is practicing in, and how to shift those: temperature, lighting, sound, color, aroma, touch, level of stimulation. Recall that our sensory organs are the main way we take in energetic qualities, so let's consider the energetics by sense organs.

Before we do that, let's acknowledge that a lot of time you may not have the ability to change the energetics of the room much. We cannot always do much about a noisy space, or facility logistics, however, we can modify whatever is possible to head in the right direction. For example, dim lighting and low tone music, may help to reduce the over-stimulation of nearby traffic. Be careful in tightly templated yoga teaching formats (e.g. Bikram, Urban Zen) in which you don't have the freedom to modify anything. There is nothing that is good for everyone all the time. Maybe you start off in some of these environments, and mature into more fluid ones in which you can really create the energetics. If this is the case, simply start with applying Ayurveda to your own life and personal yoga practice.

Sight

The lighting, colors, textures, and design are all being taken in during class. Brighter lights increase P, while decreasing K. Fluorescent lighting can increase Vata with its micromovement flickering. If instead, we're talking about bright sunlight drenched space, that can be Vata reducing (warming, natural, rejuvenative). Interestingly, dark rooms can also calm overstimulated Vata. If you are someone who uses an eye-mask to get deep rest, or destimulate, that's an example of darkness calming Vata in the mind with visual energetics.

More stimulating colors generally increase V and P, while more neutral colors decrease V and P. Warmer colors (reds, oranges, yellows, and yellow-greens) increase P quality, and decrease V and K. Cool color families (blues, grays, blue-greens) increase V and decrease P. Light and cool colors will be better for balancing K, as dark cool colors can feel like more Kapha.

Something else to consider is what the visual environment is like. Disorganized spaces increase stimulation and Vata qualities, whereas orderly spaces decrease Vata (*saucha*). Open empty cold feeling spaces (think uber modern) can increase Vata, whereas a space can be minimalist but still feel very Vata balancing if it has a lot of warm, or grounding elements (e.g. wood texture, fountains, a giant buddha statue). Too much clutter would be imbalancing for K (heaviness, accumulation), P (activated to clean) and V (overstimulating). Fresh plants and flowers, fountains, and natural elements are balancing for all *doshas*, as they are grounding, and connecting to nature. Too many different textures can be overstimulating, while too few textures can leave the environs feeling spacey—both Vata qualities.

Sound

In addition to the qualities of your speech, there are the other sounds of the Container. Music and background noise are all energetic qualities being taken in. In general, more upbeat, fast music is Vata increasing, while slower melodies and drones balance Vata. Conversely, the slow drones may increase Kapha, and the more upbeat songs could help to balance Kapha. For Pitta balancing, it's about getting them out of their heads, so mantra, chanting, or instrumental music is most P reducing. Traffic and studio noise that is distracting would all be Vata qualities. Natural sounds (fountains or naturescape soundtracks) are especially calming and balancing for V and P.

Smell

This is often a controversial modifier in Yoga. There are extremes of all practices, and generally, extremes don't serve the majority. Smoky incense tends to be balancing for Vata (heavy, musky, thick, earthy), but can be really aggravating for Pitta—especially if there are strong or artificial fragrances. Burning Sage and Palo Santo is V (earthy, smoky) and K (clearing, anti-microbial) balancing and the sweetness of Palo Santo is the best fit for Pitta. Those with Pitta imbalance are generally overly sensitive to smells, and they won't hesitate to let you know. Essential oil diffusers are less offensive to many, and we can look at the qualities and effects of essential oils for *dosha* balancing. In general V balancing oils are Earthy smelling, heavy, thick, and have relaxing properties for the nervous system (e.g. Frankincense, Vetiver, Myrrh, Patchouli, Lavender). P balancing oils are lighter, cooling, and floral (e.g. Sandalwood, Rose, Geranium, Jasmine, Neroli). Oils that stimulate circulation or alertness are K balancing (e.g. any citrus, Peppermint, Cinnamon, Rosemary).

Touch

There is personal preference here and you have to honor that for both yourself and the student. It's good to communicate openly about touch expectations. I've witnessed several teachers that offer plenty of hands-on moments ask in the beginning if anyone is uncomfortable receiving their touch (e.g. while the class is in an opening child's pose, instructing them to put their thumbs up if they would like to opt out of hands-on support). Others come around in *Sivasana* and offer everyone the same moments of minimassage. In general, announcing your touch in some way is a good way to not have the student tense up, or be surprised, or feel inappropriately touched (more likely with Vata imbalance).

Heavier pressure and longer holds are more Vata reducing. Keeping your palms pressing a student's shoulders down for a count of 10 is a good example of this, whereas a few faster massaging shoulder squeezes may help to stimulate Vata. In general, Pitta balancing is more light touch that helps them know where to focus their attention. Instructive touch (e.g. "send your breath here where my hand is touching" or "activate this part of your leg where I'm touching") feels easier to accept for Pitta predominants, and more clear for Kapha predominants. Those with a lot of Vata can feel reactive or overwhelmed with instructive touch and close attention. They do better with simply receiving the more tension-relieving adjustments.

Chart 10.3 Examples of VPK balancing shifts of the "Container"

Balancing qualities for	Vata	Pitta	Kapha
Lighting	Dim Sunlit	Dim	Bright
Colors	Warmer colors Darker colors Earth tones	Cooler colors Lighter colors Pastels Neutrals Grays	Warmer colors Lighter colors Neutrals Whites
Temperature	Warm	Room temperature	Warm or hot
Sound	Low tones Drones Slow Steady	Low tones No music Relaxing	Higher tones Faster Invigorating
Essential Oils	Earthy Floral Warming	Floral Cooling	Stimulating Warming
Touch	Announced Heavy Slow Long Tension relieving	Light Instructive Tension relieving	Instructive Stimulating

From how you speak to how you adjust, there are so many ways to modify the energetics of your offering. As the charts above demonstrate, there are infinite combinations of all of these qualities. It will be rare that you will only want to address one *dosha* in a class. I once taught a Get Ready for Bed yin-style class that was all Vata reducing. We had live tambour drone, only four to five poses total, a lot of deep breathing, supportive props, and a lot of heavy long nurturing touch. Everyone left half asleep, including me. The idea here is to give you a resource of ideas on how to shift qualities, and that you gauge how much shifting, in which direction, and in what combination, you see best.

Now that you know how to modify the energetics in your instruction, and of the Container, let's take a look at the energetics of what you cannot modify. We cannot change the qualities of the weather, the Season, or the time of day we are practicing. It is what it is. However, we can be aware of what qualities are being taken in with this larger "Container" of our yoga. Understanding the energetics of the region, which everyone is collectively experiencing, is a helpful way to know which qualities you want to shift towards, or away from.

Broader regional energetics
Seasons
Everyone feels Vata qualities (overwhelm, depletion, scattered) during the Winter Holidays, and as Figure 10.1 depicts, the qualities of time and place affect everyone in that time and place. There are some archaic rules about when Vata, Pitta, and Kapha Seasons begin and end. However, that was based on Northern India and pre-Global Warming. You can be in London or San Francisco in the middle of summer, which is typically categorized as Pitta energy, and feel cold and damp (K). While a dry, cold Winter day has typical Vata qualities, in the tropics, Winter can feel warm and damp (both opposite to Vata). In California, our seasons are shifting so that we have more typically Spring (K) weather through June, and the dry heat of the summer lasting well into October, whereas a decade ago that Seasonal cycle was shifted earlier. The point is to listen to the qualities of that day's climate, and attend to them. A class on a windy, cold Vata day could be taught differently than one on a hot and humid (PK) day—even if it's the same "Vinyasa 2" class—with all the modifications above.

Daily cycle

Another important aspect of regional energetics is the amount of daylight. Long times of darkness are more K and V, whereas prolonged sunlight is more P. If we consider an average day where there is about equal light and dark time, we'd say the early morning has K qualities (cool, damp, still, peaceful, quiet), midday has P qualities (hot, bright, active), and the evening has V qualities (cold, dark, unpredictable). In traditional Ayurveda, they demarcate the times of day as KPV, and the *doshas* also cycle through once a night. Doshic Peaks: 6am–10am K; 10am–2pm P; 2pm–6pm V; 6pm–10pm K; 10pm–2am P; 2am–6am V. Of course, daylight savings practices, and regions that don't have the average light–dark cycle, make this an imperfect science. Again, these cycles were observed by sages in ancient India. Yet, the *doshas* in the cycle of the day are quite palpable, and can be helpful to understand our energetics throughout the day. You can see why many of us have a slump around 3–4pm when P is on the decrease and V is peaking. We can also understand why spiritual practices are recommended in the early morning, during a fertile, supportive K peak. This being said, the most heating and intense yoga *asana* is best balanced in this early morning K time, and would be too heating for midday, and too depleting during the evening. A moderate, steady, part strengthening and part relaxing practice would be good for P time, and a rejuvenative, yin-style practice great for the evening. We often see intense and active classes slotted at that afterwork V time, yet this is a time when we are supposed to be getting ready for rest and unwinding. Similarly we find lunchtime power workouts in the middle of a P peak because it suits modern professional schedules. We may not be able to circumvent these market driven factors in class schedules, but we can be aware of the energetics, educate our students, and make some small adjustments. Below, I walk through some case studies that include these dynamics.

Astrological cycles

Of course, we can get fancy and also incorporate larger energetic forces such as moon phases and planetary shifts (e.g. Mercury retrograde, or Solstice). The Moon, Sun, and planets are large energetic bodies, and we do experience their energetics (think of Seasonal Affective Disorder, menses, ovulation), just as we take in climate and seasonal energetics. However, this is advanced.

Making your modifications palatable to your demographic

It's great that we can be aware of the energetics on so many levels—*asana*, our instruction, the Container, and regional energetics. However, our students may not be. And they may not care. The corporate executive coming in for a Core Power class in her lunch break may not care that its the peak of P time, and that she's aggravating her obvious Pitta imbalance; she just wants to sweat and get her workout done in an efficient manner. If you try to lead a purely Pitta reducing class for her, she may walk out, complain, or stop attending. Commonly, we're going to have find a way to reconcile the students' desired energetics with what we know is more balancing. It's just like sneaking vegetables in kid cuisine—a lot of kids don't like veggies, but as parents we want them to not fuss about eating them, so we get a little crafty sometimes. Ultimately reconciling conflicting needs and shifting energetics on the fly, is an art, just like getting in as many veggies as you can without shifting the taste so much that kids reject the dish.

Give them some of what they want, and some of what they need.

Case study 1

Let's take that corporate executive lunchtime yoga case and play with how applying some shifts could look. In order to fulfill her goal to get a workout in and sweat, we can include some longer held poses to build intensity. The increased duration also gives time for adjustments, which make her feel like she's optimizing (P loves optimizing). We can include a few more challenging modification options and transitions to make her feel like she really worked hard. All of the above are P qualities that she is seeking.

Now, because of her energetics, and the time of day, and how much P is already in the style of class, our consideration is how to bring in some opposite qualities. There are infinite ways we can shift qualities, but here are a few approaches that could work well in this case:

- Build up the intensity of the poses and then slow down, so the class has a crescendo and decrescendo. This allows us to use the beginning and end to do more grounding, stretching, relaxing, and less heating poses.

- Start off with seated neck, shoulder, or facial stretches. This gets her grounded right away, and she's hitting her high tension areas and happy about that. Progress into hip stretches because we know she's seated most of the day in computer posture. Because these are her tight areas, she feels like she's being productive right from the beginning, even though the effects are Pitta balancing.

- Offer some anatomical focus, but also bring in feeling based focus in cueing. The anatomical cues are important for her to feel like she can trust your instruction, and be more open to the feeling based cues.

- Have her close her eyes, and cue her to do this as challenging modification (which it is in all standing *asana*). Bringing the gaze inward (*pratyahara*) helps to decrease mental activity and balance Pitta. If she feels this is an additional challenge, she'll be drawn to this modification. It's also a nice way to decrease the Pitta in those standing poses in the peak of the class intensity.

- Similarly, we can add in cooling breathwork in challenging poses, or resting ones. Lion's breath exhales are great to release heat in challenging poses, while lunar breath would be easier to do in the more restful poses.

- She's unlikely to have the patience for a long rejuvenating *Sivasana*. So, instead, bring deep hip stretches and long twists, all on the ground in the decrescendo of the class. These poses decrease Pitta and give her some relaxation time at the end, despite the shorter *Sivasana*.

- A water fountain is a super easy and simple background Pitta reduction.

- Positive feedback and acknowledgement are important for all humans, but those with a lot of Pitta especially. They are naturally really hard on themselves (self critical), and less likely to celebrate their achievements than to see where they still need to improve. By providing positive feedback, we help to assuage the effects of their inner critic.

Case study 2

Let's do another case with married, retired women, almost all with excessive weight. They're attending a late morning class almost as a social activity and are more interested in chatting and drinking tea than working out. Sometimes they show interest in learning more philosophy and emotional balance but for the most part aren't incredibly motivated. Despite the lack of drive, they're incredibly consistent in attending. In this case, we've got a whole lot of Kapha going on.

Again, if we gave them a purely K reducing class, they would find it too challenging. So, we'll make sure that we incorporate some K to give them what they want. Some great ways to do this would be: to encourage knees down and taking rests; allow time after class to connect with you; share aspects of your personal journey during class; and a class playlist that at least begins and ends with some grounding music. These women are just as much there for connecting socially as they are to practice. Allowing them to connect with you fulfills this K need. Sharing aspects of your life, philosophy, or practice when relevant accomplishes this during class. Having a firm boundary to connect after class, instead of before, ensures that you start on time, and maintains your energetic state before teaching. Remember, while sharing your journey can be endearing, it can also be annoying, ego-driven and alienating if you overdo it, or you don't allow for understanding of others' realities. Preaching veganism, Hinduism, celibacy, politics, or preaching anything is *not* what I'm suggesting. The most relatable parts of your journey will be how you experience your yoga journey, and what you are learning.

Now, for our crafty modifications to decrease Kapha for these lovely ladies:

- Fast build-up of intensity, then plateau, then come down, then build-up again, then come down. In contrast to the classic crescendo-decrescendo arc, this approach accomplishes a few K balancing shifts. Keeping the intensity up for the first half of class (e.g. Vinyasa, dynamic movement) gets the hard part done and doesn't allow them to double think it. While the intensity is on the higher side, it's not so challenging that they are unable to do what you are instructing. Push them to their limit, which may be lower than a classic high Pitta student. The midway decrease in intensity is an important break to not overwhelm them. The second build-up in intensity could be great as core work on the ground, or other core strengthening poses that are a bit slower paced. We want them to feel a bit less intensity than the first half of class, but still increase their heart rate.

- Start standing. It doesn't let them get too grounded and heavy before they start moving.

- Vinyasa and dynamic movement in *asana* are great ways to increase K balancing qualities.

- Invigorating breathwork is another great way to increase the intensity, or K balancing in the second peak/ second half of class. Bhastrika, or Kapalabhati breath—slow and steady—are great options while kneeling.

- Aromatherapy is generally more accepted by high Kapha folks, especially when they have a longstanding relationship with you. Offering optional aromatherapy at the beginning of class, or using a diffuser are both easy ways to bring in some activating, stimulating scents.

- I mentioned above having more grounding music at the beginning and end of class; however, in the middle of class we can bring in more upbeat and happy, light music (lyrics are fine) to balance K.

Private sessions

All of the above information can be used for attending to the energetic needs of your private clients. With private clients, there are additional opportunities to tailor energetics. Generally speaking, we have a bit more freedom to shift the qualities of the student's experience.

Bring in opposite qualities to what they feel

We can customize sessions a bit by their Current State. You're not an Ayurvedic practitioner, and it will help you to emphasize that to manage their expectations (and to cap the amount of time they're talking). By simply emphasizing qualities in your inquiry, you can get a good sense of where they are at. Here are some examples of "check in" questions to get a sense of the qualities and *doshas* they are feeling and needing:

- How have you been feeling recently?
- Where do you feel stress in your body?
- What kids of things are you feeling in your body?
- How's your sleep?
- How's your tummy and digestion feeling overall these days?
- What qualities would feel really good to you today?

The specific words you use don't really matter. Any line of questioning that gets them to express some of the qualities they are experiencing will work. The more general, the better. When you get specific, it tends to lead to stories and extraneous details. Pay attention to the words they use in their response. Categorize them as qualities and *doshas*, and focus on bringing in the opposite.

Modifying energetics in the interaction

Next, we can consider the energetics of your interaction with the client as a professional. Is the interaction loosely defined (e.g. they just call you when they feel they need a session), or is it structured (e.g. you meet at the same time each week)? The more variability there is, the more Vata there is, for both you and the client. If you have a high Pitta client, they are likely to want to initiate scheduling and will be drawn to goal-oriented approaches. That means that you don't have to stress structure, but rather offer them what you'd like to achieve with your work together over X number of sessions.

Most high Kapha folks don't initiate private sessions—they prefer to be without such focused attention. However, they are able to honor regularity and structure. With them, standing appointments may be easier, and best in the morning. Also, changing what you are doing and how you are stimulating their bodies is a good thing for balancing K. Of course, you'll want to bring in those changes in an easy, non-drastic way—maybe keeping the same starting/ending for each session and then shifting the focus on different parts of the body in between.

High V clients likely won't be able to stick to the structure you have, but the structure benefits both of you. Here, you may want to stress purchasing a session package to encourage them not floating away from your work together (they still may), and don't take it personally when they doubt their decision. For additional V balancing, try to keep the sessions around the same time of day, or the same day of the week, or at least in a rhythm (e.g. weekly). Being firm on boundaries and on the structure is a good thing for them, but don't be surprised if they are reactive at your not making an exception for a 24-hour cancellation policy, or them being 30 minutes late. Just smile, listen, and emphasize that you need to be loving to yourself. With so much Vata going around, and the entitlement that generally comes from people that have the money to pay for private sessions, these situations are common. Remember that you are a professional, and this is your business, and that you don't need clients that bring in energetics that are not beneficial for you.

Summary

- *Asana*s have some inherent energetic effects, which can be modified based on how they are practiced.

- You can shift the energetics a student experiences by consciously choosing the qualities of your instruction.

- The energetics of the space we practice in are significant and modifiable.

- When choosing how to modify, we can consider the *doshas* in season, time of day, climate, and demographic.

- With private sessions, there is additional opportunity to modify qualities, and customize.

Appendix 1: VPK in My Life Worksheet

WHAT ARE THE ENERGETIC PATTERNS IN MY LIFE?

We'll focus on the qualities of the experience in your life *now*, so we can see which *doshas* are predominant in these aspects of your life at present. We'll go further into this in the next chapter, when we look at your Current State.

Naturally, as humans, we are biased. That's okay. Bias is irrelevant because it's honored as the natural state of things. That we each perceive our experience uniquely is a central tenet we'll explore later. In Ayurveda, all that matters is how *you* experience the energetics of the various aspects of your life.

Out at a restaurant for a meal with a friend, I may bring in more Vata than my companion. I felt stimulation, movement, overwhelm, and frenetic energy. My friend felt relaxed, nurtured by the food and my company, and well taken care of by the restaurant staff. Irrespective of what my friend experiences, the energetic input for me was Vata because the qualities I felt were all Vata qualities. For my friend, it was a more Kaphic energetic input because all of the qualities of her experience were Kaphic.

- Consider how your experience of each of these areas of your life *feels*; not what you *think* it is, or want it to be. For example, our experience of food can feel irregular, changing, extreme, and overwhelming even though from the outside looking in, we may seem to be "health conscious" eaters.

This worksheet is available to download from www.ayurvedabysiva.com/worksheets

- It's also perfectly normal to have a varied experience. A relationship can feel nurturing and grounding as well as inconsistent and depleting. When you have the qualities of more than one *dosha* present, you have more than one *dosha* present. It's just that simple.

- The next step is to get a sense of which qualities/*doshas* are present a greater percentage of the time in that experience, as this will reveal which *dosha* is predominant in that energetic input for you. If the relationship is more often nurturing and grounding (Kapha), than inconsistent and depleting (Vata), then Kapha is the predominant energy in my relationship.

- This is for you and only you. There is no "should" here, and no judgement. Well, it's natural to judge what you find, but try to replace that with the perspective that *you are here for a reason, and it's for your greater health, emotional wellbeing, and spiritual growth.*

Work (includes home-making)

Consider the pace, the movement, the people, the workspace, and the work itself.

Food

Consider the tastes, textures, and your experience of cooking and eating.

Relationships

Pick one to start, a major one. It doesn't have to be a partner, just the person you spend the most time with. Consider both the qualities of the person and of the relationship—you're absorbing both. If I have a mother that is very nurturing by nature (K), but our relationship is up and down and unpredictable (V), then I'm taking in K and V, and which qualities I feel *more of the time* are going to reveal the predominant *dosha*.

Routine

Think about the flow of your day, your sleep-wake cycles, the pace, the movement, the rhythm.

Appendix 2:
Constitution Survey

The idea behind this survey is that if you answer several questions about your genetically determined body features, and your long-term patterns across several systems, we can get a sense of the doshic ratio in your Constitution.

This does not replace the assessment a practitioner can provide, but is a good proxy, and a great place to start getting to know yourself from a doshic perspective.

Please read these few tips, for a more accurate experience:

- Remember the *spectrum of human features*. You may think you have a big nose, for example, or big nose for *your* face, but think about the spectrum of noses in the human race and where the size of yours would fall in that spectrum.

- Think about how you were when in your *younger years*. For example, you may feel like you have thin hair now, but if it was thick in your younger years, that's a more accurate depiction of your Constitution.

- Think *long-term* for the patterns, like over decades, or your whole life; not just the past few months or years.

- You can have features in *more than one* column; CHECK ALL THAT APPLY.

- You don't have to have every feature listed to check a box. If it *feels like you* in some part, check it.

This worksheet is available to download from www.ayurvedabysiva.com/worksheets

Category	Vata expressions	Pitta expressions	Kapha expressions	
Body structural features				
Eye shape	smaller size; darker color e.g. brown-black, grey	deep set; medium size; brighter color e.g. bright blue, green, hazel, orange flecks	large size; thick lashes; more protruding eyeballs; deeper color e.g. deep blue, chocolate brown	
Gaze	constantly shifting; feels like you may have your attention elsewhere to others	penetrating gaze; direct; intense; good eye contact	soft gaze; not intense but present; heavy lids that may be half closed	
Nose shape	small; narrow; crooked	straight on profile; angular; medium size	large size; wide base; large nostrils; rounded tip	
Space between eyes	narrow	medium; protruding	wide	
Lips	thin; wrinkled; dry; brown or grey	medium; pink; bleed easily	thick, full; smooth	
Face shape	long, oval; thin	angular, squarish	round; full; high cheek bones	
Teeth	thin; irregularly shaped; crooked; ridged; discolored grey	medium size; yellowish; tend to cavities	large size; smooth; white	
Neck	long; curved; prominent adam's apple	medium; muscular	short; rolls of skin; double chin	
Body structure	tall; lanky; long limbs; not very muscular; thin	medium height; muscular build; toned	short; stocky; wide; curvy; round or squarish	
Bone structure	thin	medium	thick and solid	
Hair	thin; wiry; tight curls; frizzy; dry; black, dark brown;	medium thickness; bright; blonde, red; oily; straight	thick; lustrous; wavy, loose curls; oily	
Subtotal	**Vata**	**Pitta**	**Kapha**	

Category	Vata expressions		Pitta expressions		Kapha expressions	
Long-term body function tendencies						
Appetite	fluctuating; get full quickly; tend to not really ever get physically too hungry and can just graze; forget to eat; get lightheaded or dizzy without food		strong; irritable and angry if not fed; need meals and snacks; need full meals to stay full		low; could eat one meal a day; no am appetite; like to eat sweets late at night	
Sleep patterns	light sleep; frequent night waking; restless		tough to turn the mind off to fall asleep; solid sleeper; alert upon waking; wake before alarm; hot at night		love being up at night alone; tough am wake; foggy mind in am; thick heavy sleep	
Skin patterns	dry; flaky; discolored; dull; T-zone combination skin on face; blackheads		red undertone; prone to inflammation/ irritation; pimples; rash prone; oily		smooth; oily; deep cysts or blemishes; whiteheads	
Body temperature	usually feel cold; cold hands and feet; crave heat		usually feel hot; heat intolerant		neither extreme; prefer cool climate but adapt easily	
Speech patterns	effusive; exuberant; tangential; fast		clear; direct; logic based; point driven		slow; don't say much	
Subtotal	**Vata**		**Pitta**		**Kapha**	

Category	Vata expressions	Pitta expressions	Kapha expressions	
Mind and emotional core features				
Personality traits	artistic; charismatic; interested in the "new"; love to stay busy; need to travel; embody extremes; low follow through; lots of ideas; impulsive decisions; changeable	natural leaders and teachers; love to learn about how things work or why; tend to be more cerebral than emotional; ideals and "shoulds"; detail oriented; concerned with efficiency, productivity, cost-effectiveness; read consumer reviews; logical decisions	mellow; more quiet; stay in jobs, homes, relationships for long; don't often initiate; hesitant to change; passive; prefer supportive roles; hold deep attachments to people and things; loyal; good listeners	
Long-term mind and emotion tendencies				
Adaptability	high; in fact usually the cause for need to adapt is a change in your mind/decision	fair; okay to change course or decision with good reason; intolerant of flakiness	low; prefer to stick to the plan or not shift; take a long time to get comfortable with change	
Response to stress	get overwhelmed/intimidated and escape; perhaps never really address the problem and stay distracted	great; do well under pressure; come up with solutions and resolve the problem	withdraw and isolate; need to be alone to contemplate or insulate with food/sleep	
Subtotal	Vata	Pitta	Kapha	
Total	Vata	Pitta	Kapha	

Appendix 3: Signs of Imbalance Chart

This chart lists out common symptoms across tissue systems. It's not all-inclusive, but rather focused on symptoms and tissue signs that you can feel on your own, i.e. without labs or professional diagnostic measures.

This does not replace the assessment a practitioner can provide, but is a great place to start listening to what your body is conveying about "where am I at?"

Please read these few tips, for a more accurate experience:

- Focus on the now. The now is a bit ambiguous because it really means your feeling of "now." For some of us this could be the last few days. Others of us will feel like we've been in a similar place for the last few years. I'd suggest not getting caught up on the time distinction and simply noting what feels present in your tissues.

- You may have multiple symptoms in the same part of the body. More signs and symptoms mean a greater degree of the *dosha* present. So noting how many of the symptoms you have is valuable.

- You can have features in *more than one* column; CHECK ALL THAT APPLY.

- Tally up the number of symptoms you noted in each of the areas of the psychospiritual body (Emotional Body and Mind sections).

- Tally up the number of symptoms you noted in each of the areas of the physical body (Digestion to Reproduction).

Category	Vata signs deficiency, irregularity, degeneration	Pitta signs inflammation, infection, heat	Kapha signs accumulation, stagnation, congestion, growth	
Emotional body	overwhelm anxiety and worry hypersensitive extreme emotion internal conflict cycling emotions	irritable impatient short-tempered angry jealous resentful	sad want to be alone psych. baggage holding on to grudges depression crying	
Mind	Reactive trouble sleeping indecision restlessness difficulty focusing difficulty completing racing thoughts impulsive choices addictive tendencies	intense focus on problems activated to solve overworking pressured to-do list mania overanalyzing (self) critical impatient righteous	unmotivated unclear dull stubborn unmotivated tough am wake	
Non-physical subtotal	Vata	Pitta	Kapha	
Digestion	gas, gurgling, bloating belching cramping, spasm constipation dry, small stools straining low appetite	hyperacidity increased appetite > 2 BMs/day loose stools narrow stools mouth sores	sluggish digestion poor am appetite low physical hunger mucus in stool nauseous in am heavy after eating	

Immunity and blood	low immunity allergies food sensitivities cold hands and feet feeling cold headaches—vasospasm		feeling hot flushed face, ears headaches—tension gout herpes outbreaks Inflammation tendency		not temperature sensitive elevated blood sugar swollen feet/hands	
Skin	dry, flaky discolored, dull blackheads dry, itchy skin dry cuticles		red undertone inflamed red acne rash or hive prone		smooth oily whiteheads deep acne cysts	
Sinuses and respiration	dry, cracked lips dry sinus membranes runny nose dry throat dry, itchy eyes		sinus infection bloody nose/mucus respiratory allergies		congestion am phlegm post nasal drip clogged ears headaches—sinus pressure	
Nerves and adrenals	trouble sleeping dark circles under eyes		spend a lot of time in "get-it-done" mode		slow responses over sleepy weight gain	
Muscles, joints and mobility	pain stiff creaky joints worse in am tremor unsteadiness in movement		inflamed muscles and joints worse after use		swollen ankles swollen, cool joints joint pain with rain slow movement	
Kidneys and urination	urinary frequency		frequent urinary tract infections		bladder/kidney stones cloudy urine	

cont.

Category	Vata signs *deficiency, irregularity, degeneration*		Pitta signs *inflammation, infection, heat*		Kapha signs *accumulation, stagnation, congestion, growth*	
Sexuality and reproduction	extreme sexual frequencies and practices after time, no libido dry tissues irregular menses uterine cramping		frequent yeast infections with burning STDs		slow to rise libido sluggish orgasm excessive discharge yeast infections with fewer symptoms heavy menses dark, clotted menses fibroids, polyps ovarian cysts enlarged prostate	
Physical subtotal	Vata		Pitta		Kapha	

Appendix 4: Current State Survey

This blank chart offers a structure to your regular self check-in. Use your own words to describe the qualities and symptoms you feel in the various parts of you.

Then, add up the number of symptoms and qualities you noted for each *dosha* to get subtotals. These subtotals are just a quick proxy for revealing the relative degree of *doshas* present within your tissues. Rather than focusing on an exact sophisticated analysis, I'm offering a tool for quick and broad insight into your Current State.

The Additional Reflections will help you prioritize which *doshas* should be attended to most in your balancing efforts.

Category	Symptoms and qualities present	*Doshas*
Emotional body		

cont.

Category	Symptoms and qualities present	Doshas
Mind		
Subtotal	Non-physical body	V P K
Additional reflections	Which *dosha* is there the most of? Which *dosha* has been around the longest? Which *dosha* is causing me the greatest bother?	
Digestion		

Immunity and blood		
Skin		
Sinuses and respiration		

cont.

Category	Symptoms and qualities present	Doshas
Nerves and adrenals		
Muscles, joints and mobility		
Kidneys and urination		

Sexuality and reproduction		
Subtotal	*Physical body*	V P K
Additional reflections	Which *dosha* is there the most of? Which *dosha* has been around the longest? Which *dosha* is causing me the greatest bother?	

Appendix 5: Balancing Check-In

ASSESSING IMBALANCES

1. Do I have signs of imbalance? Which *doshas* are involved, and where?

Use your Signs of Imbalance Chart and/or your Current State Survey.

2. What are the *sources* in my life of this energy? (Try to identify at least three.)

Correlate with *VPK in My Life Worksheet* (Appendix 1) if you'd like.

1. Which imbalances are the *most*, or have been around the *longest*?

2. Bonus: Any imbalances seem *secondary*?

Hint: Secondary imbalances come *after* signs of other imbalances had been in those tissues for a while already.

BALANCING APPROACH

1. What *qualities* would be opposite, or balancing, to what you feel in your *emotions*? And in your *digestion*?

2. Can the *source(s)* of the imbalance be targeted?

If you can't really eliminate the source of an imbalance quickly or easily, try to shift the qualities within the experience—like bringing in plants and calming music to a Vata work setting. If you're stuck, bring in the opposite qualities in other ways in life—like Vata reducing diet to offset the Vata work setting.

1. *How* can you bring in *opposite qualities*?

Simply brainstorm any ideas that come to mind. If you're stuck on what is opposite, just ask: What qualities would make the symptoms you have feel better? *Anything* that allows you to *feel* the opposite qualities counts!

1. Bonus: Which are the *easiest* changes to bring in?

We all have our ideas of what is going to be best or most effective, and our society prioritizes that in decision making. Here, I'd love for you to prioritize based on ease, or lack of resistance. Why? Well, because we could all use more ease. And second, so you can start feelings some shifts sooner. The easiest shifts are the ones you'll stick to most, and consistency breeds momentum.

Appendix 6: Self-Reflective Exercise

Pick *one* shift to bring in for digestive balance, for at least two weeks.

This could be a Vata reducing approach to food. It could be being still and present while you eat. It could be a shift in what you are eating. Anything!

But please, limit yourself to *one* shift. It's easy to go for two. I want you to experience what just one feels like—simple, loving, present.

One way in which I'll bring in opposite qualities
of my imbalance in digestion:

This worksheet is available to download from www.ayurvedabysiva.com/worksheets

Appendix 7: Self-Reflective Exercise

1. Identify an area of life where you are experiencing some unpleasant feelings.

2. What do you feel are some of your unmet emotional needs in the situation?

3. If magically, those needs were met, how would you feel?

4. What are other moments, memories, or ways in which you can get yourself to feel the same feelings you listed above?

References

Frawley, D. (2006) *Ayurvedic Healing Course for Health Care Professionals, Part II.* Santa Fe, NM: American Institute of Vedic Studies.

Ganesan, U. (2010) "Medicine and modernity: The ayurvedic revival movement in India, 1885–1947." *Studies on Asia Series IV, 1,* 1, 108.

Makary, M.A. and Daniel, M. (2016) "Medical error: The third leading cause of death in the U.S." *British Medical Journal 353,* i2139. Available at www.bmj.com/content/353/bmj.i2139, accessed on November 01, 2018.

Sainath, P. (2018) "India's agrarian crisis has gone beyond the agrarian." *The Wire,* 2 July.

Saini, A. (2016) "Physicians of colonial India (1757–1900)." *Journal of Family Medicine and Primary Care 5,* 3, 528.

Shunya, A. (2017) *Ayurveda Lifestyle Wisdom.* Boulder, CO: Sounds True.

Villoldo, A. (2015) *One Spirit Medicine.* Carlsbad, CA: Hay House.

Further Reading

Chopra, D. (2001) *Perfect Health*. New York: Bantam Books.
Chopra, D. (2015) *Quantum Healing*. New York: Bantam Books.
Chopra, M. (2015) *Living with Intent*. New York: Harmony Books.
Frawley, D. (2009) *Inner Tantric Yoga*. Poole: Lotus Press.
Klein, M. (2017) *Kitchen Ritual*. Los Angeles: Pranaful.
Shunya, A. (2017) *Ayurvedic Lifestyle Wisdom*. Louisville: Sounds True Inc.
Silcox, K. (2015) *Happy Healthy Sexy*. Hilsboro: Beyond Words Publishing.
Tiwari, M. (2001) *The Path of Practice*. New York: Ballatine Books.
Villoldo, A. (2015) *One Spirit Medicine*. London: Hay House UK.

Index